MOODTOPIA

Molly,
Thank you so much
for allow me to teach
About Breastfeeding!
Happy to share my
passion of herbs!

Scott :)

MOODTOPIA

Tame Your Moods, De-Stress, and Find Balance
Using Herbal Remedies, Aromatherapy, and More

Sara-Chana Silverstein, RH (AHG), IBCLC
with Susan K. Golant, MA

Da Capo

LIFE
LONG

Copyright © 2018 by YourHERbalist Inc.

Hachette Book Group supports the right to free expression and the value of copyright. The purpose of copyright is to encourage writers and artists to produce the creative works that enrich our culture.
The scanning, uploading, and distribution of this book without permission is a theft of the author's intellectual property. If you would like permission to use material from the book (other than for review purposes), please contact permissions@hbgusa.com. Thank you for your support of the author's rights.

Da Capo Press
Hachette Book Group
1290 Avenue of the Americas, New York, NY 10104
www.dacapopress.com
@DaCapoPress

Printed in the United States of America
First Edition: August 2018
Published by Da Capo Press, an imprint of Perseus Books, LLC, a subsidiary of Hachette Book Group, Inc.
The Da Capo Press name and logo is a trademark of the Hachette Book Group.

The Hachette Speakers Bureau provides a wide range of authors for speaking events. To find out more, go to www.hachettespeakersbureau.com or call (866) 376-6591.
The publisher is not responsible for websites (or their content) that are not owned by the publisher.

Print book interior design by Linda Mark

Library of Congress Cataloging-in-Publication Data
Names: Silverstein, Sara-Chana, author. | Golant, Susan K., author.
Title: Moodtopia: tame your moods, de-stress, and find balance using herbal remedies, aromatherapy,
and more / by Sara-Chana Silverstein, RH (AHG), IBCLC with Susan K. Golant, M.A.
Description: First edition. | New York, NY: Da Capo Lifelong Books, 2018.
Identifiers: LCCN 2017060943| ISBN 9780738220048 (paperback) | ISBN 9780738220055 (ebook)
Subjects: LCSH: Anxiety disorders—Alternative treatment—Popular works. | Herbs—Therapeutic use—
Popular works. | Self-care, Health—Popular works. | BISAC: HEALTH & FITNESS / Herbal Medications. | HEALTH
& FITNESS / Alternative Therapies. | HEALTH & FITNESS / Aromatherapy.
Classification: LCC RC531 .S4748 2018 | DDC 616.85/22—dc23
LC record available at https://lccn.loc.gov/2017060943

ISBNs: 978-0-7382-2004-8 (paperback), 978-0-7382-2005-5 (ebook)

LSC-C

10 9 8 7 6 5 4 3 2

To my mother, Enid Natalie Bluestein, who loved me passionately and gave me the strength and self-confidence to know I could accomplish anything I put my mind to. May she have an immediate Refuah Shleimah.

CONTENTS

Contents

PART IV
Pulling Yourself Together

PART I

Moods: Can't Live with Them,
Can't Live Without Them

CHAPTER ONE

FACING THE CHALLENGE

Life is a train of moods like a string of beads; and as we pass through them they prove to be many colored lenses, which paint the world their own hue, and each shows us only what lies in its own focus.

—RALPH WALDO EMERSON

MY OLDEST DAUGHTER WAS SUBSTITUTE TEACHING AT A PRESCHOOL WHEN I received a call from her just as I was getting ready to work out at the gym.

"Mom, it's so weird," she said, sounding a little worried. "My right arm is tingly and numb, and I just don't feel right."

"Do you want me to pick you up, or can you take the subway home?" I asked.

"Why don't you come get me?" she replied. An independent millennial, this was so unlike her. I quickly changed back into my street clothes and was reaching for my car keys when she called again.

"Now my left arm is numb," she reported.

"Call an ambulance," I advised, breathless now from anxiety. "I'm on my way."

As I arrived, the EMT informed my daughter that she hadn't had a heart attack or a stroke. This news was not greeted with joy. "A stroke?" she said incredulously to the EMT. "Of course, I didn't have a stroke. I'm twenty-seven years old!" We called our family doctor in Brooklyn, and he told us to come straight to him. Together, we'd decide how to proceed.

My daughter slowly walked to the car, and I drove to our doctor. The numbness continued unabated, and within two hours, she had lost all sensation in her body from the shoulders down. She had become a quadriplegic. After three weeks in the hospital, the prognosis was that she would be bedridden for the rest of her life. Her doctors gave up on her and were preparing to send her to a nursing home where she would spend the rest of her life. Oh. My. G-d.

The doctors diagnosed that she had transverse myelitis, a neurological disorder caused by inflammation of the whole spinal cord that severely and (usually) irreversibly damages the nerve fibers. An acute form of this disorder can come on within sixty minutes, and sadly, this was my daughter's diagnosis and prognosis. How could this have happened? After many false starts and turns down blind alleys, the best we could figure was that, because a few months earlier she'd been hit by a tow truck, the accident might have caused an undetected blood clot in her spine.

I am the mother of seven children. Over the years, I'd learned to balance my parenting duties with my full-time career as a master herbalist, classical homeopath, and lactation consultant. But now, I had to set aside my former life and spend nearly four months living at the hospital 24/7 with my stricken daughter, after which we were transferred to a rehab facility for three more months.

I'd made a vow that I would stay positive with my daughter, but I was finding it impossible those first few weeks. This was the most challenging time of my life. Some days, when I would leave the hospital to buy us food, I wouldn't even look both ways when crossing the street, in the secret hope that I'd be hit by a car and be put out of my misery. Other times, I just wished I could open the window on the twelfth floor of her hospital room and throw myself out. To see my daughter unable to even scratch herself if she was itchy or wipe her eyes when she cried was too much for me to bear.

Before this tragedy, I'd been organizing my thoughts for this book. I'd spent many years helping women understand their emotions. I'd taught them how to empower themselves rather than drown in their feelings, and here I was, facing what surely must be the most difficult test a human could endure, and I felt I was failing. I was a hypocrite. I would duck out of the hospital room and bawl in the stairwell so loudly that the sound reverberated off the walls. With no hope to be found, I was a disaster . . . I hadn't slept in two weeks, couldn't eat, and could barely speak. I would collapse on the bathroom floor down the hall, unable to breathe, my body convulsing in sobs.

But then, one day, Nurse Rita showed up. No . . . she didn't come to our rescue—or maybe she did, but in a backhanded way. You see, Rita was nasty; Rita was negative; Rita was sour. I wasn't even aware of how kind and wonderful the other nurses were until I encountered one who was mean. But she did do something right: she lit a fire under me. I decided that even if I didn't make it through this test, I would muster the courage to help my child. I would help her find her strength so that she would stay positive and in control of her emotions rather than getting lost in the moods that this horrible injury had created. I made a decision to not let my feelings dominate my actions. I would rise above them. I would create an environment of healing for my daughter.

First, I'd had enough of grumpy nurses like Rita and frustrated doctors who treated my daughter as if she were a "hopeless case," so I hung a huge sign on the door of her room saying, "You can only enter if you're smiling and nice." I barred access to anyone who would bring negative energy. I discovered what time the nurse in charge picked the staff for the following day and demanded that my daughter receive care from only those who were upbeat and surrounded her with positive energy.

Next, I decided to "fake it" with my daughter since she wasn't in a position to handle my reactions—and it was unfair for me to foist them on her. After throwing up in the bathroom from grief, I would clean myself up and then walk into her hospital room with a grin on my face. I helped her respond to her friends' texts and e-mails. They starting arranging delicious meals for us. We became proactive. (Okay, I did cave sometimes. I am only human, after all. But I worked on it.)

I changed whatever I could in the hospital environment. I didn't touch the monitors and medical equipment, but no one considered what my daughter needed to feel safe—so that was something I could do. For instance, I moved the bed and furniture around so she could immediately see who was entering the room. I sprayed different essential oils daily so we didn't have to smell the sad odors of the hospital. I purchased fresh flowers every day and taped get-well cards on the walls from her friends and hand-drawn pictures from their kids. I found the funniest photo in *Vogue* of high-fashion boots that looked exactly like the heavy medical ones she had to wear to prevent her feet from getting stuck in one position. We got a hoot out of that.

I bought her T-shirts and leggings in her "color palette" so she looked stunning every day. The colors really made her feel better. I washed and brushed her hair and polished her nails with her favorite color. I found a little garden area outside and brought my daughter there in the wheelchair when the doctors finally allowed me to take her out. Every frustration pushed me to find a positive solution. Every no I heard from the doctors, I changed into a maybe as I became the foremost authority on transverse myelitis.

And as for self-care, the smile on my face (even if it was plastered on), essential oils, pictures, flowers, colors, and positive energy helped me, too. I also took herbs every day to soften my sadness and anger. Certainly, my herbs couldn't fix the problem, but they helped temper my reactions.

After our first two months in the hospital, I realized that I was incorporating into my handling of this crisis all the tools I'd planned to write about in this book. The best part was that they were really helping my daughter and me. I began coping in ways I'd never thought possible. The guidelines I share here kept me together enough to enable me to encourage my daughter to heal. I was able to hold my emotions steady (not always, but at least most of the time), and I was able to learn which doctors I could cry to and which were turned off by tears. I learned how to control my anger unless I could use it to get my child what she needed. In fact, while I had been working with women on stabilizing their moods and emotions for years, I learned more about moods and emotions in those eight months than I had in my whole life before then.

The best news is that by the time I was able to start writing, my daughter was defying all odds and predictions. Rather than being bedridden and paralyzed for the rest of her life, she is now out of the hospital on her way to a full and complete recovery.

She's a hero. And I'm a survivor.

WHAT IS MOODTOPIA?

Moodtopia means being in control of your moods so they don't control you. Plain and simple. It means being able to identify your mood, acknowledge that it's real and okay, but also decide whether it works to benefit you and those around you in any particular moment. It doesn't mean being euphoric or happy all the time—that's an impossible and actually unwanted goal! But it does mean having greater awareness about your moods and how to manage them.

Facing the Challenge

Although you may never encounter the dire circumstances I did with my daughter, most likely you will find yourself in a stressful situation that can trigger moodiness. We all do! In fact, emotional extremes are part of what makes us human—they're hardwired into our brain and our hormonal system . . . they help us bond with our children, decode what our partner is feeling even before a word is spoken, empathize with those in need, and communicate passionately.

Our feelings are a large part of what makes us tick. They are real and true. But after spending decades helping women, raising my own children, and being a woman my-self, I know that moodiness is a problem for many of us. It's a question that comes up when I work with teens, new moms and dads, grandparents, and even little girls and boys. Sometimes our feelings get the better of us. Whether or not it's hormonal, we can find ourselves crabby and irritable. We're short-tempered and easily triggered; passionate and intense. We get hijacked by our anxiety or anger and suddenly we're out of control, yelling at our children, acting spitefully toward our mother, or sulking in a corner . . . resentful and even bitter over a girlfriend's snub or a sister's unkind remark. Unfortunately, these negative emotions as well as the darker energy that leaks out of us at these difficult times are destructive not only to our own well-being but also to the happiness of the people we love.

These strong feelings arise at all stages of our life. We all know about the moodiness of the "terrible twos," and let's not even get into teenagers' mood swings! Although women often attribute moodiness to their menstrual cycle, we all know that the nonhormonal times can be just as emotionally challenging.

Most individuals who struggle with moods feel they've either experienced or are currently suffering lots of stress. Anxiety and tension change the way your body functions chemically and how your mind responds emotionally. But there are many actions you can take to help you. Taking herbs, for instance, pampers, supports, and nourishes your body and brain. Herbs can help end the cascade of negative chemicals that flood you when you're frazzled. And when you stop this cascade, you can ultimately learn to be in control of your moods so they don't control you—a state of Moodtopia.

My intention in writing this book is to help you find your own Moodtopia. We all handle our moods uniquely. Some of us hold them in and get stomachaches and headaches; some act out; and others seem contained but in actuality are like pressure cookers ready to explode. On the other hand, some of us should be handed awards because we've figured out how to handle our waves of emotions and express them appropriately. We know that stress is a real ingredient to poorer health outcomes as we age. We need to ask ourselves: Is the situation we're in so stressful that it warrants the flood of emotions we're feeling? Or are the emotions we're expressing more problematic than the situation at hand? If we could learn to understand our emotional responses and feel more in control of them, would we then feel less stressed? More balanced? I believe we would.

Now this may seem like an impossible goal because, as we all know, bad things do happen to good people and everyone has cruddy days, cruddy months, and even cruddy years. A good cry, shrieking like a banshee, wanting to throw a plate across a room, or yelling at other drivers through a closed car window is appropriate more often than one would expect. But I also believe that as we battle through this crazy world, we need to be able to gain control of our moodiness. The best way to do this is with awareness.

With some thought, insight, tools, and effort, we can harness these negative feelings and use them to our benefit—and not let them get in the way of our happiness. From my experience with thousands of clients, I have learned that most of us have not been given the skills to recognize these feelings or prevent them from dominating us. Although this moodiness factor is inborn in all of us, in our fast-paced culture today, it's hardly attended to. So, despite our best intentions, our roller-coaster emotions are infectious, spreading to the people we least want to hurt, leading people around us down a rabbit hole of angst and distress. And who wants that?

HERBS AND MORE TO THE RESCUE

Moodtopia will give you the understanding, the observational skills, and the tools to change your life in just three months! The information in this book will allow you to be the master of your emotions. It will show you how to approach your moods from unique perspectives, from understanding the "Cycle-of-Sanity" to identifying and relying on your intuition, to seeking help from medicinal herbs, to attending to the colors you wear, and the way you decorate your home. This multidimensional approach has been very successful in my practice with thousands of women over the last twenty-five years. And it's what helped me and my daughter extricate ourselves from the depths of our darkest moments.

Facing the Challenge

As I mentioned, I am a master herbalist RH (AHG), classical homeopath, and board-certified lactation consultant (IBCLC). I am also a TV and radio health expert, keynote speaker, businesswoman, wife, and the mother of five boys born in close succession and two girls. (Yes, I have a lot of energy!) For over twenty-five years, I've worked with nearly twenty thousand women, helping them achieve the healthy state they desire, guiding them on how to give birth naturally, teaching mothers to successfully and painlessly breastfeed their babies, and most important as relates to this book, helping them deal with mood swings that can disrupt the peace in their home.

I see clients over the course of their life—often two to four times a year as a complement to their relationship with their family doctor. So many today want to approach their ailments naturally and to support any medical treatments with holistic remedies. Just as I successfully provide the latter to my patients, I can also help you find alternative ways to deal with your emotional ups and downs. *Safe and proven medicinal herbs may be just what you need to help you improve your life not only for your own well-being but also for the sake of those you love.*

WHAT YOU CAN EXPECT

The healing path and specific cures in *Moodtopia* are based on the treatments and steps I teach and suggest to women in my practice. It encompasses many dimensions—physical, emotional, and spiritual.

In truth, there's a gap between feeling anxious and blue and needing antidepressants, antianxiety pills, or other mood-related medications. Here's where herbs step in. They're a gentle, natural way to enhance your emotional state and nourish your nervous system so you can withstand the stresses of modern life without the potential unwanted side effects medications can have (although I do not oppose them since I've seen that, for some, they can be lifesavers). Indeed, if you are struggling with depression and/or serious anxiety, panic attacks, and other psychological issues that last more than a few days, herbs can be a life-enhancing relief. But if you don't see improvements with the herbs, then it's important to seek the advice of your doctor, therapist, psychologist, or a master herbalist, since clinical depression can be dangerous. And, if you are taking any medications, check with your health-care provider before taking herbs, for any contraindications.

The first steps of my program involve awareness. You'll learn about the "Cycle-of-Sanity" that will help you appreciate the recurrent nature of your feelings. I'll also ask you to document under what circumstances your moodiness arises. Once you are aware of your unique triggers, you can improve your disposition by following suggestions you'll find in the rest of the book.

After you've prepared yourself emotionally this way, in Part II, I'll first show you how to prepare your body physically by supporting your liver and using "adaptogens"—agents that help calm your overall reactions to stress. They'll keep your system running smoothly and allow you to thoughtfully use the many herbs and aromatherapy suggestions in this section to help alleviate stress and quiet negative emotions. By the way, aromatherapy is the use of essential oils that, in therapeutic doses, promote physical, emotional, and spiritual health.

In Part III, you'll find additional, essential complementary tools—your Moodtopia bag of tricks. There are many avenues to follow. Try the ones that appeal to you because they'll help you attain insight, be more self-actualized, and empowered:

+ Faking it—putting your best face forward
+ Learning to recognize and trust your intuition
+ Understanding positive and negative energy so that you can identify people and places that make you feel bad as well as those that make you feel good. This can mean finding your healthy, positive energy sources.
+ Creating a protective bubble so you can shield yourself from destructive energy forces
+ Relying on color to soothe and create a sense of serenity

Finally, in Part IV, I provide you with a 90-day step-by-step program to incorporate many of my suggestions. You'll find recipes for snacks that give you a lift when your energy is low and charts that organize the remedies I suggest by issue. This is your Moodtopia Program.

I have made hundreds of suggestions in these pages—all of which I fully stand behind. But don't feel intimidated or believe that you have to adopt this plethora of information to banish your moodiness. I'm sure you'll find several ideas among the many that you resonate with. These are the ones to turn to when you're feeling stressed and out of sorts. They will help you.

. . . . ⚜ . . . .

Taken together, my advice can help turn moodiness and a sense of feeling overwhelmed into cheer and calmness. And with an attitude of fun and adventure, you—and everyone around you—will flourish.

FALLING MADLY IN LOVE WITH HERBS: THE MAKING OF AN HERBALIST

When I was a senior at the University of California, I was invited, through a Yale University drama program, to study Shakespeare and Chekhov at Oxford University. England! Hurray! But while my fellow students were happily analyzing these literary titans, I could be found sitting on the floor of the local health food store, poring over *Back to Eden* by Jethro Kloss and *Common Herbs for Natural Health* by Juliette de Bairacli Levy—definitely not what Yale had in mind.

Why had I become so interested in herbs and healing? I'd had severe childhood allergies; I survived on allergy shots and antihistamines. The allergies continued to plague me through young adulthood, and once again I found myself struggling, but this time I was far from home and my regular doctor. There had to be a better way to treat my allergies, so I turned to the massive Oxford library and my love of research to look for answers.

These authors presented a different way to look at medical problems. They advocated using herbs, breathing, walks, and healing massage. Absorbing what these books had to offer, I realized that it was possible for all of us to heal ourselves and our family with plants. I understood that the world had within it all the healing properties we would ever need.

In my tiny dorm room at Oxford, I began making decoctions of herbs. Glass jars filled with floating flowers, leaves, twigs, and roots were lined up on my desk. As I took herbs, my allergies started getting better, my sleep improved and my overall energy was more consistent. Over the next few years, back in the United States, I pursued the artistic life as a ballet dancer, and the herbs I continued to take relieved muscle pain and kept my muscles strong. I felt a big difference in my performances.

Ten years after my awakening to botanicals at Oxford, I found myself sitting in a class on herbs in Manhattan with a group of New Age hippies from all over the tristate area. They all lived in rural communities. I took the train in from Brooklyn in my high heels and coral nail polish, with my sunglasses perched on my head—not your typical herbalist. I was there to learn as much as I could to help myself. One thing stands out in my mind from that time. During one of her lectures, our teacher said, "If you want to heal someone, just see what grows around their house."

Oh no, I thought. I live in Brooklyn. What do we have? Fire escapes, exhaust fumes, concrete, and dog poop? Nothing grows where I live. I spoke to the teacher after class and told her I thought her comments didn't apply to my situation. She threw *The Peterson Field Guide to Edible Wild Plants* into my hand and said, "Walk around your neighborhood and open your eyes."

I grabbed my husband and begged him to join me in a walk. Within the first two blocks around my building, we found ten medicinal herbs. Like the rose in Spanish Harlem, they were poking out of cracks in the concrete in alleys, along the curbs under parked cars, in rain gutters, and through crevices in building foundations. They were all around me, if I'd only pay attention!

It wasn't long after this class that I became a mom and soon found my children dealing with serious allergies that the pediatrician couldn't control with standard medicines. I turned to herbs with new commitment and the wise herbal treatments of a neighborhood Traditional Chinese Medicine (TCM) practitioner. To my amazement, what my allopathic doctor could not cure in my daughter, my Chinese herbalist could. She no longer needed a tissue in her hand at all times, she stopped snoring like a truck driver, and the bags under her eyes began to recede. Her skin returned to a rosy glow, and her eyes sparkled. When my second child was born with eczema and began a similar wheezing-and-chronic-stuffy-nose pattern, I knew that I had to study herbal medicine and homeopathy professionally. I began a five-year homeopathic training program and upon graduation, I plunged into my training in botanical herbal medicine. In the end, I completed five years of homeopathic and two additional years of herbal training. During this same period, I also became an international board certification lactation consultant, logging in 2,500 clinical hours of breastfeeding training.

DISCOVERING THE EMOTIONAL-HEALING PROPERTIES OF HERBS

Until my children were born, I'd used herbs for purely physical issues. I'd learned that botanicals helped lower blood sugar, increase thyroid function, support the liver, and reduce high blood pressure. But I never believed they could soothe emotional issues until I experienced it myself.

When I first learned about the herb motherwort, I was intrigued but dubious. It could reduce my gloominess? Really? So, I decided to try it on myself. When I became crabby and took motherwort, the gray cloud that was ready to envelop my body and flip my mood dissipated in twenty minutes. I was able to rationally articulate what I was feeling and shed the skin of a helpless victim of my emotional state. What a revelation! I learned to anticipate what would make me moody . . . if I was going to be in that kind of situation, I would run for the motherwort. As I did more research into the world of botanicals, I started using other herbs to modulate my moods. As a result, I was able to communicate better and be a calmer parent—especially as the mother of seven children.

Imagine this scenario: At three forty-five each afternoon, my five sons would burst into our small apartment punching, yelling, throwing their clothes on the furniture, dropping their cereal all over the place . . . letting off steam after a tough day at school. But instead of screaming at them, I would take a dropperful of an herb called skullcap and chill out. I didn't grit my teeth, my stomach wasn't in knots, and I didn't explode because my floor was covered with smashed crackers, books, and jackets. Skullcap is my go-to herb for stress. It wouldn't change the reality of what was happening around me—no, boys will still be boys. Rather, it changed how I *reacted* to the noisy chaos. The motherwort and skullcap helped me get through those times with more grace and aplomb than anyone could have reasonably expected.

I realized herbs could benefit the women in my growing practice as well. My many interactions with my patients taught me their issues were often multidimensional. Although they were coming in for a breast infection or their child's chronic ear infections, their moodiness seemed a more pressing issue. I knew that with my herbal education, I would be able to help them gain better control of their emotional states. I started to apply to the women in my practice the mood-healing remedies I developed for myself. I began educating them about which herbs were available. Much to our shared delight, my clients' moods improved appreciably. And they were happier mothers and wives, sisters, and neighbors for it.

Remember, herbs will not fix or change the situation that's creating your nervousness, stress, or anxiety. But they will help calm your system, make you less reactive, and allow you to find better ways to problem-solve. The remedies you'll find in Part 2 of this book are the same ones I've been recommending for decades to those who come to me for help. Over the course of the years, I learned that if people are taught about their predisposition to moodiness at an early age, they'll realize this is normal and just the way they are hardwired. And if they are also taught the skills needed to control their moods, including the use of herbal remedies, they'll feel empowered to establish attainable emotional goals and not feel victimized by the ebb and flow of their own internal states.

I AIM TO show you how you can manage your moodiness and negative feelings when you find yourself at the threshold of your own emotional prison. From my experience with thousands of women and my own family's trauma, I have come to see that moods are to be respected and honored. I know that the teachings in this book will help you overcome moodiness and go on to a happier and more peaceful and productive life. But at the same time, I also know that in the right context, negativity has the potential to drive positive actions. That being true, I will show you how using your moods can also lead to impassioned actions that make positive changes in the world.

My hope is that after reading *Moodtopia*, you gain skills that will help you feel more stable in this very unstable world and walk away with tools that will allow you to be super emotional when *you* want, and learn how to hold in your emotions if that is what's best for the situation. Learn how to honor your moods and be in control to create the life you want to have.

My favorite saying is: "We're not in charge of what happens to us in life, just how we respond to it." That was certainly true with my daughter's spinal cord injury, and it's still true today for all of us.

CHAPTER TWO

UNDERSTANDING THE "CYCLE-OF-SANITY"

My recipe for dealing with anger and frustration:
Set the kitchen timer for twenty minutes, cry, rant, and
rave, and at the sound of the bell, simmer down and go
about business as usual.

—PHYLLIS DILLER

REMEMBER WHEN I WAS RAISING MY BIG FAMILY, AT LEAST ONCE A WEEK I would throw back my head and cry, "I have never been this sad/upset/angry/frustrated/anxious/[you name it] before!"

But my kids would chuckle and say, "Yes, you have, Mom. Remember last week?"

Whenever an intense feeling or mood would present itself, it would feel new to me when, in fact, it was part of my typical, habitual, and predictable cycle of emotional reactions. Ironically, my kids were better observers of my behavior and moods than I was!

We live life on a continuum of emotions. I like to envision it as a circle. We start with happiness—the state we all want to be in. However, it's clear that no one ever stays happy all the time. Something frustrates us, and we then move into sadness or anxiety, or anger, or the blues. In a typical day, we go through all these emotions repeatedly. This is a normal and even helpful process, and what you'll learn is that it's always cyclical. It's the way the world was created—the seasons cycle, the moon cycles, our bodies cycle. This cycling creates movement, and movement is healthy.

For instance, we know that when fluids are stuck in our physical body, we become sick. We begin with a cold, but if the mucus stays too long in the nasal passages or the lungs, we develop a sinus infection or bronchitis. The lack of movement caused by inflammation of joints can prevent fluid from circulating there, contributing to arthritis. With such a condition as varicose veins, the blood cannot travel back to the heart easily, it becomes stagnant, and when it stays too long, pain begins. The same thing with constipation: when stools stay in the large intestine for too long . . . well, I don't have to tell you how that person feels.

Our emotions work in the same way. New York City acupuncturist Anton Lee, MS, LAc, explained to me about how Korean medical theory frames this issue. "Energy flows through our body like a network of 'roads,'" he told me during an interview, "almost like a highway system. Our emotions can block the free flow of energy in the body like when a highway is under construction. Or if an accident occurs, traffic not only backs up close to the accident but also on secondary roads that feed into or out of the affected area. This is true in the body also. Our emotions can cause blockages in different places all over our bodies."[1] When our feelings get stuck in this way, it's hard to maintain our emotional health.

That's why I teach my clients about the "Cycle-of-Sanity." I have found that with this understanding, we can begin to have more control over our moods.

A TALE OF FORTY COATS

Here is a typical situation when living within the "Cycle-of-Sanity." As a California girl transplanted to New York (not by my choice, by the way), I get very frustrated when fall approaches. Although I love the leaves as they change color and begin to blanket the streets with gorgeous burnt oranges, burgundies, yellows, and browns, I begin to worry about coats.

Yes, coats! I have raised seven children in a tiny Brooklyn apartment, and each of my kids has minimally four coats. Every child has one coat for windy days, one rain jacket, one stylish going-out coat, and a parka for when the temperature dips below freezing and the wind howls. So, with nine of us in the house (including me and my husband), that means I have to organize and find places for a minimum of three dozen coats of varying sizes and thicknesses. By September, I grow uneasy at the thought of taking down all the coats that have been beautifully and neatly assembled on storage shelves that I'd had built up high, close to the ceilings of the apartment. I spend days begging the weather not to change. I read and reread the weather reports, hoping for a sudden heat wave that would last from October to June. But no matter how much I pray and beg, the temperature on the East Coast begins to drop and panic sets in as I keep asking myself, "Where will I find room for thirty-six-plus coats without clogging up my house?"

So now I feel *frustrated*—I mean very frustrated. Every little thing begins to get under my skin. And lo and behold, my frustration turns into *agitation* and *anger*, and I start an internal monologue that begins with, "I never wanted to move to New York in the first place. If we lived in Los Angeles, each of us would only need one jacket, maybe two, tops!" I begin saying to myself, no matter how silly it may seem, "I really can't handle this challenge. It's too much for me! How can I make space for these jackets when there's already no space in the apartment? I can't stand it!"

So, what happens next? I become *melancholy*—miserable, gloomy, and withdrawn.

Then, one Monday afternoon, while sitting in the dentist's office waiting for one of my kids to finish having his teeth cleaned, I see a women's magazine. I flip through it, and there it is. A unit that attaches to the wall with forty-five hooks for jackets. Now I have this *insight* that if I purchase this unit and nail it up in the entryway to my home, I will have a place for all the jackets and maybe even a few extra spots for guests' coats. I have the profound *insight* that I can handle this perennially irritating situation, and since I have found a way to *problem-solve*, I suddenly feel *happy*!

I've made it all the way around the Cycle-of-Sanity and come out on top again. Hurray!

· · · · · · · · ## A Few Words About "the Blues" ·
and Clinical Depression

Having the blues (being sad or even melancholy) is different from clinical depression. The blues is characterized as everyday sadness that arises from recent, external, difficult events, such as injuries, illnesses, work setbacks, or the loss of a loved one. It's situational and will ease in several weeks as you make your way around the Cycle-of-Sanity. Clinical depression is another animal altogether—some have described it as a soul-crushing sense of futility and despair that doesn't go away. A person with clinical depression ruminates on the negativity (with repetitive worrying, brooding, and self-defeating thoughts), thus reinforcing it. *Clinical depression requires medical attention because it can lead to suicide or other self-destructive behaviors.* According to Los Angeles psychologist Dr. Mitch Golant, here are some of the most common symptoms:

BODY:

Physical pain

Insomnia or sleeping too much

Nightmares

Loss of appetite or overeating and binging

MOOD (which may or may not be linked to external events):

Dullness and boredom; lethargy

Loss of interest in favorite activities

Loss of sexual desire or insatiable desire

Self-loathing

Angry outbursts

BEHAVIOR:

No energy to carry out everyday tasks

Uncontrollable crying

Withdrawal: No capacity to get out of bed, get dressed, shower, or take care of other personal needs, such as eating or going to work[2]

. . . . ⚜ . . . .

SEARCHING FOR AN EPIPHANY

As I discovered a solution to my coat conundrum and made it back to happiness, I learned something profound. Real happiness comes from *insight* and being able to *problem-solve.*

Understanding the "Cycle-of-Sanity"

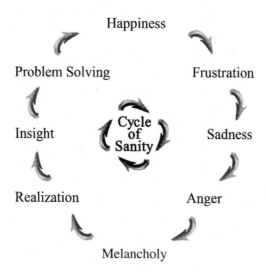

When we are challenged with a certain situation, as soon as we have an insight about it, we already begin to feel better. In fact, I believe that for most people, simply being happy isn't as rewarding as emerging from more negative emotions with that "Aha" moment. That's what actually feels good. When I sit with a client for an hour and a half as we discuss a challenge she's struggling with, I usually see the biggest smile when she suddenly looks up at me and says, "Now I get it! Now I know how to solve this problem." It's liberating and empowering to have the insight that leads to understanding.

Everyone craves this part of the cycle. Insight is even more exciting than happiness. If you think about all the great philosophers and scientists across centuries, it was insight they were searching for. The understanding. The epiphany that made their lives worthwhile.

But here's the good news. We don't have to have very deep revelations to get that "Aha" feeling. No, we don't have to have the answers to such questions as why water feels wet, or where the universe ends, or what the meaning of *meaning* is. We just need such thoughts as "Oh, so that's why my toddler is so clingy!" or "Now I understand my husband!" or "This is how I'm going to manage too many coats!" It's the small epiphanies that really keep us going. Once you understand what needs to be done, you can solve any problem.

Wouldn't life be easier if every time you felt frustrated, you knew that in the end you would have an insight to help you resolve the issue? That way, you could actually accept and even welcome your frustrations—instead of feeling angry or sad about them. But what if your frustration teaches you there's nothing you can do about the situation? That's also an epiphany. And here it is:

Why waste your precious energy on something that has no solution?

Time to let go.

FOLLOWING YOUR FEELINGS

So, does life always cycle? Yes, for most people, the Cycle-of-Sanity happens all the time—every day of every week and every month of every year. I want you to observe and recognize these daily cycles in your own life and not be afraid of them—and I'll help you do that in the next chapter. Feel free to replace the feelings I've charted with your own—it doesn't much matter what you call them. Just know that this is how we all function.

The more you can understand the circularity and see it in your life, the easier it will be for you to control your moodiness. When you feel that first burn of frustration and truly understand that right around the corner, you'll have an insight that will lead to problem solving, you'll keep better control of your reactions. If you can honor the emotions as they arise on the right side of the circle and be aware that this is normal and that you'll soon be able to go through the understanding on the left side, then you'll become the master of your moods.

FIGHTING SELECTIVE AMNESIA

Every single human being, no matter what culture or country he or she comes from, experiences all of these emotions: happiness, frustration, agitation, anger, sadness, and melancholy in the same cyclic way. But like me, when these feelings finally pass, we suddenly develop amnesia and forget that we'd ever had them.

Moody people often think in extremes: *"This is the worst thing that's ever happened to me!" "I've never been so hurt!" "I'm so angry I can explode!"* As you'll see, these emotions are neither good nor bad. Rather, they're real and true and part of how we were created. To know this gives you power. I wish that children in preschool, elementary, junior and senior high school, and even college were taught to appreciate all of their feelings—the good and also the so-called bad ones. Most people are ashamed of their deep emotions and don't realize that most of us experience them. They can feel isolated, scared, and intimidated as they believe that something is very wrong with them. They try to hide their emotions, or squash or repress them, and as a result, they get moody. But these feelings are part of human nature and can actually be good for them.

So, let's look at the hidden positive aspects of the emotions we usually want to push aside.

·········· The Secret Benefits of Negative Emotions ·················

+ **Benefits of frustration:** Often we feel powerless when frustrated, but the experience doesn't have to be negative. Frustration is positive when it propels us forward. We can allow this aggravation to either hold us back or push us toward action. Sometimes we have to become really frustrated to generate the energy needed to make a change. Without this irritant, we could remain stuck in a situation that's hurtful for us. That's why frustration must be honored and applauded. If we use it properly, it's often followed by amazing results.

+ **Benefits of sadness:** Paradoxically, sadness is positive because it can fill us with appreciation for what has been good in our lives. It can help us treasure those special moments and render us more caring. Having experienced sadness also gives us the ability to feel compassionate toward others who've gone through or are going through what we are. It can connect us to them more deeply and open us to receiving their help. And it can fill us with appreciation for the times we don't feel sad.[3]

+ **Benefits of tears:** Emotional tears also contain more mood-regulating manganese than do the other types. Stephen Sideroff, a clinical psychologist at UCLA and director of the Raoul Wallenberg Institute of Ethics, explains that stress "tightens muscles and heightens tension, so when you cry you release some of that because crying activates the parasympathetic nervous system and helps restore the body to a state of balance."[4]

+ **Benefits of anger:** Anger brings a lot of power with it and can be a motivating force that allows us to accomplish things we couldn't if we remained more passive. It can give us the push to defend the underdog and combat what feels like aggressive forces that can be blocking our success. Acknowledging anger and not trying to suppress it can help lower stress on the heart and manage pain. Expressing anger as it arises, instead of bottling it up and then letting it all out in one explosive blast, can help us tame its intense power. Perhaps more than anything else, anger benefits us by *alerting us* that something is wrong and needs action. Indeed, being in denial is often more dangerous than anger.

+ **Benefits of the blues:** The blues have the ability to stop you in your tracks and push you to take action, because like physical pain, they're a signal that something wrong needs fixing. The social withdrawal that sometimes accompanies melancholy can help people examine issues in their life that are not working. Being alone is not "bad." It can give you time to really understand where the sadness came from and what your next step should be. The blessing is that once you've gone through tough times, you can come out the other end stronger and more resilient. This gives you the experience to be able to help another person to endure the same situation. As such, then, singing the blues is really a gift.

. . . .

GETTING STUCK AND UNSTUCK

We need to move around the Cycle-of-Sanity because problems can arise when we stay in one phase for too long. When we literally get "stuck" in frustration or anger, these usually normal and beneficial emotions can go haywire.

It's hard to be around people who are stuck in one area of the Cycle. After a while, it becomes too difficult to remain close to a person who's always frustrated by every little thing. You can try to be sympathetic, but how long will your patience last? You may have lots of compassion and be supportive of someone who's sad, but if sadness stretches on and on, it may be hard for you to continue to be encouraging. Anger is certainly called for in certain situations, and as we've seen, it also has a positive side because it can create the energy of change. But to hang out with a person who's chronically angry is very stressful.

We think of being stuck in negative emotions, but mental challenges can begin if one becomes stuck on the more positive side of the Cycle, too. It can boggle the mind to be with someone who's in a constant state of insight. Those incessant "Oh-my-G-ds" can drive you nuts! And, sad to say, it's also concerning if a person appears to be constantly happy. So, our goal is understanding that emotions come and go, and that they and this cycling are normal. We need to honor them and stay emotionally fluid, flowing from one feeling to the next effortlessly. Think of being graceful as a ballerina with your emotions as they rise and fall.

In fact, one of the best ways to help you free yourself from stagnant and stubborn negative feelings is to start moving—yes, exercise. No, you don't have to be a ballerina and you don't have to commit to an aerobics class—but you can park a few blocks from your destination or take the stairs or run with your kids or pull weeds or even do some strenuous housework. Much has been written about the benefits of exercise on moods—it releases endorphins, our body's natural painkiller, in the brain.[5] Sebastian Plettenberg, master Gyrotonic movement instructor in New York, told me that often his clients will come in with physical complaints—a stiff neck or backache—but once they start moving, they realize that an unaddressed emotional issue has been behind their physical discomfort.[6]

My work with my client Julie demonstrates how complex being stuck in an emotion can be. And it also shows how wonderful and life-affirming it can be to get "unstuck." Julie had been depressed for many years but her antidepressant drugs weren't helping her. Willing to try other modalities, she came to me for homeopathy to treat the depression. I spent almost two hours with her and suggested daily fifteen-minute walks coupled with a homeopathic remedy. On her way home, she purchased the remedy and took it before she went to bed. The next morning, she woke up feeling very agitated. She called me to ask what to do. I told her to be patient. Next, she called me because she was crying. For hours and hours. She was crying so much, her husband had to come home from work as she was unable to care for their kids. Then, she got very angry—with me. She called me, saying, "I will never take another homeopathic remedy ever again!" Ouch!

Six weeks later, my office manager informed me that Julie had made an appointment for a follow-up visit. Honestly, I was scared to see her again, knowing how emotionally disruptive this remedy had been for her.

She waltzed into my office, calmly plopped herself onto my couch, and began her story. "I really felt low for a few days after my crying spell," she told me. "But when I pulled myself together, I started walking like you suggested. In fact, I walked right to my office to quit my job. I've been working for the same boss for ten years, and he didn't treat me with the kind of respect I feel I deserve. He made me work overtime night after night. I couldn't leave for a couple of hours once or twice a year to watch my kids' performances in the school play. He never complimented my commitment to my job and hasn't given me appropriate raises along the way. I was fed up."

But she didn't actually leave. As Julie was tendering her resignation, her boss begged her to stay. "I told him I would only remain if he changed ten things—and I handed him my list. He agreed, and I kept my job. But it's on my terms now. And I know I can quit later if I feel he hasn't kept his side of the bargain. It was so empowering."

Next, Julie withdrew both of her kids from the private school they were attending. She'd always hated it and had only enrolled them there because her in-laws had insisted. She registered them in the school she had wanted them to be in all along. Then, she dug into the family savings account and put down a deposit on a larger apartment. She had moved into her husband's bachelor pad when they had first gotten married, but now, with two children, they were on each other's neck all the time. They could hardly breathe! She realized that her husband had issues with change and would never get up the guts to move, so she just did it! She looked at me with awe in her eyes and said, "How did I get the confidence to do this?"

· · · · · · · · What Is Homeopathy? ·

In 1796, Samuel Hahnemann created homeopathy, an alternative medical system based on the principle that "like cures like." It can be an effective tool in alleviating moodiness and works by moving energy that gets stuck when a person has emotional challenges. Herbs, on the other hand, enter the bloodstream and physically alter emotions and responses to stress. The wrong homeopathic remedy will have no action in the body. But with the correct remedy, the client will feel a shift, though it may take a while to rebalance oneself.

Homeopathic remedies are made from plants, flowers, minerals, or bacteria. During their production, the chosen substance is diluted and then shaken repeatedly in a process called being *succussed*. The liquid is then poured over sugar pellets, which absorb it. These are placed in a vial and labeled. On the bottle, you will find the name of the remedy, such as "Ignatia," plus a number and letter. The numbers range from 6x, 6c, 12c, 15c, 30c, and 200c, to 1M and 10M. These correspond to the remedy's potency and represent how many times it was diluted and succussed. With homeopathy, the philosophy is that the more a substance is diluted, the stronger it becomes. So, diluting it two hundred times makes it stronger than diluting it six times.

A homeopath suggests a remedy only after taking a person's "case." A typical consult lasts from one to four hours; the homeopath's goal is to understand the client's unique needs.

. . . . ⚜ . . . .

In homeopathy, we believe when given the proper support and environment, the body is a self-healing mechanism. The homeopathic remedy gave Julie's system the push it needed and the exercise increased her energy and helped loosen her mood. Without these changes, she couldn't work through her depression—she was stuck there. Her mind could only heal, her depression could only begin to pass, she could only move to the next phases on the Cycle-of-Sanity, if she had the strength and confidence to have insight (I hate my job; I hate my kids' school; I hate this apartment), which then propelled her to problem-solve. "I haven't felt this happy in years," she told me. She learned a great lesson: there are actions she can take when she gets into a depressive state. She went back on her antidepressants, and remained in maintenance mode, taking a lower dose of the drugs with her psychiatrist's approval.

We spent the next few sessions going over the Cycle-of-Sanity. We discussed how Julie could be aware of this cycle, and she understood that these emotions were normal and safe and they would pass if she were more fluid in her life and willing to go through the steps to get to the problem-solving stage. We also discussed how her frustration and sadness were not "bad" emotions. Rather, they were alerting her to situations in her life that needed to be changed. She saw that with a few important adjustments, she could get out of her rut.

I know that Julie needed that homeopathic remedy to help her do what she needed to do to get unstuck. Homeopathy helps people move energy. I also told her that a good cry can sometimes be a magic tool in allowing a person to get to their next step.

Another client, let's call her Debbie, came to me for chronic urinary tract infections (UTIs). In taking her case, I referred to *Materia Medica*, a resource for homeopathic practitioners and herbalists that lists thousands of remedies. I typed her symptoms into the search engine, and a famous homeopathic remedy usually given to angry people kept coming up for her. I was confused. She was one of the sweetest and gentlest women I'd ever met. Well mannered, friendly, kind. At first, I was hesitant to give her this remedy, but after having input the data several different ways, I was sure this was what she needed.

After eight weeks, Debbie called to report that for the first time since she could remember, she was UTI-free. But she wanted to come in again. She, too, plopped herself on my couch and started to recount her story.

"I've been so angry for the past couple years," she explained, "but didn't know what to do about it. It's my mother-in-law. She has severe emotional problems. One day she's nice to my kids [who were 6, 8, 12, and 14], but the next she'll yell at them. She's so unpredictable. I've been angry because my husband is in total denial. He doesn't know how to handle her; he never speaks about her; and he pretends her inconsistency isn't a problem. I feel so sorry for my kids. They don't deserve to be yelled at. I made this appointment with you because even though my UTIs are better, I still don't know how to handle my mother-in-law. But at least, I feel ready to take action now."

We decided the best way was for her to take each child aside individually. She would look her children in the eye and have a frank, age-appropriate discussion with them about their grandma. Using this strategy, Debbie would support her kids the way they needed to be held, and they, in turn, wouldn't feel that their grandmother's rage was directed at them personally. Debbie had her "Aha" moment, could let go of her buried anger, and move along the Cycle to problem-solve. This allowed her to regain her physical health.

ADDICTED TO EMOTIONS

I remember learning about the healing properties of the herb tobacco. When we students heard the words *healing use of tobacco*, everyone's mouth dropped open in shock. But our teacher explained that tobacco has been used for generations in Native American tradition for religious ceremonies. The traditional view is that "sacred herbs are powerful, but when misused or disrespected, their power consumes us. Tobacco can be a healer or a destroyer. It depends on how and how often it is used. When used in a sacred way, it can promote good health and assist with spiritual guidance and growth."[7] On the other hand, when inhaled without the sacred overlay, tobacco takes control of the smoker, and he or she becomes addicted.

The same is true of our emotions. They are normal. They are natural. If we were taught that we should embrace frustration because it will help us grow, or that sadness is part of life and that we'll experience it from time to time, or that anger can push us to make changes in our lives, we'd all view our moods in a very different light. If we expect that these emotions just come, that they are part of us, that they will resolve when we allow them to—if we think of them as gifts—they can become holy.

On the other hand, if we pretend that we're not supposed to have negative feelings and don't accept them graciously and with honor, they, like tobacco, can rule us and take over our lives. Can people get addicted to frustration, sadness, or anger? Yes, I believe they can.

One of my forty-year-old clients, let's call her Jacklyn, had always fought with her mother, whom she would call once, maybe twice a day. They would yell, and Jacklyn would become mad and sad and frustrated. I made a deal with her to help her break this destructive pattern. I told her that she could come stay with me for a weekend—with one caveat: While she was with me, she was not to call her mother. I would check in with the older woman twice a day to make sure she was safe, but Jacklyn was not to call her for three days.

For the first twenty-four hours, Jacklyn was calm. When she asked to call her mother, I said, "No way. We had a deal." On day two, she snuck into the bathroom, called her mom, had a fight with her, and walked out of the bathroom, bumping right into me. (Remember, it's a very small apartment.) I was scowling at her. It was then that I realized that just like a heroin addict, Jacklyn was really and truly "addicted" to the rush she got from arguing with her mom. It was a habit that had turned into an addiction. She couldn't go more than twenty-four hours without a conflict. She had become a rageaholic.

As we spent time working on this, Jacklyn realized that not only did her mind need these fights, but so did her body. Dr. Candace Pert's research teaches us that "a feeling sparked in our mind-or-body will translate as a peptide being released somewhere. [Organs, tissues, skin, muscle and endocrine glands], they all have peptide receptors on them and can access and store emotional information." This means emotional memories are kept in many places in your body, not just or even primarily in your brain. "You can access emotional memory anywhere in the peptide/receptor network in any number of ways," Dr. Pert continues. "I think emotions are literally lodged in the body."[8]

Can an emotion create a flow of chemical reactions that we become addicted to? Yes, they can. Certain emotions, and especially stress, have been shown to create physical symptoms similar to those that come from addictive illicit street drugs, such as cocaine, crack, ecstasy, and methamphetamines: increased heart rate and blood pressure, increased blood sugar, lack of focus, breakdown of muscle tissue, difficulty multitasking, and disengagement. In addition to the hormones adrenaline and noradrenaline, stress also releases dopamine, a "feel-good" chemical. This is responsible for addictions other than drugs, such as gambling, shopping, and sex. Dopamine encourages repeat behaviors by activating the reward center in our brain. It has been shown to be at the heart of many addictive behaviors and substance abuse issues.

As for Jacklyn, even before we could start herbal therapy, she had to see a psychotherapist. She was totally unaware that she had been addicted to the adrenaline rush that comes with anger because it felt so normal to her.

What to Do If You Feel You're Addicted to Certain Emotions

Some of the herbs discussed in Chapter 5 can help you break the addiction, but you may also need professional help. I especially recommend craniosacral work discovered by Dr. John Upledger and biophysicist Dr. Zvi Karni. Their research led to the discovery that the body often retains (rather than dissipates) physical forces and the accompanying emotional energy, triggered by physiological, psychological, emotional, or spiritual trauma. Craniosacral therapist Elizabeth Poole, PhD, explained the underpinnings of this work to me this way: "Many healing modalities have described that pain caused by unresolved emotions or physiological, psychological, spiritual or birth trauma or shock can lodge in the body. Craniosacral therapy is particularly effective in relieving pain and in assisting in the resolution of the primary cause of that pain, be it physical or emotional...."[9]

GAINING CONTROL BY LETTING GO

Becoming aware of the Cycle-of-Sanity and how it works is the first great step in gaining control of your moods. Now, assuming that you don't have more severe emotional issues, such as clinical depression, bipolar disorder, or borderline personality disorder, and aren't stuck in a certain phase or addicted to rage or other difficult feelings, what are the next steps you can take to flow smoothly from one phase to the next?

Let me begin with a story drawn from Jewish folklore.

It's said that famous King Solomon, who lived from 970 to 931 BC, was wise and powerful beyond measure. Yet he complained to his advisers, "I am too depressed in my life. When everything goes my way, I am afraid that it won't last. When things do not, I fear that my woes will never end. I've had a dream that there is a ring which contains the knowledge to give me peace of mind. Go and find that ring for me. I wish to have it by Succoth [a holiday celebrating the harvest], six months from now."

His advisers searched the world over, each asking for this powerful ring that would bring the king peace of mind. They went to the finest jewelers, the richest lands. Finally, Succoth approached. Since no one had ever heard of such a magical ring, all of the advisers gave up—except one . . . the youngest of the group. He found himself walking restlessly through Jerusalem all through that last night. As morning dawned, he found himself in a very poor district. An old man was setting up a stall with simple jewelry and trinkets for sale. In one final desperate attempt, the adviser described the ring and King Solomon's request. The old man thought for a while. He took out a plain gold band and began to engrave something on it. Then, he handed it to the adviser. As the young man read the script, his heart leapt with joy. "This is it!" he shouted.

That evening at the Succoth feast, the king asked his advisers whether they'd found the ring that would solve his problem. Most stood by silently, their heads hanging in shame, as they had failed in the quest. "We have!" spoke the youngest, surprising everyone. He came forward and placed the ring on the king's finger. The king looked at the ring and read the Hebrew words engraved there: *Gam Zeh Ya'avor*, "This too shall pass."

As he read, the king's sorrows turned to joy, and his joys to sorrow, and then both gave way to peace. The king was reminded in that moment that all his riches and glory were impermanent, and all his sorrows would pass away as did the seasons and the years. From that time on, King Solomon wore the ring and remained in a peaceful, balanced state—Moodtopia.

Can you repeat the mantra: "This too shall pass"? I know it's very hard when you're in the middle of difficulties, but it's true. One truth I can say for certain: living in the world as we know it today, the only thing that's truly constant is *change*. Everything is transitory.

This age-old wisdom exists in other spiritual and religious contexts as well, including Buddhism. Here's how this discipline frames the advice: A student went to his meditation teacher and said, "My meditation is horrible. I feel so distracted, my legs ache, I'm constantly falling asleep. It's just atrocious." The master answered matter-of-factly, "It will pass." A week later, the student came back to his teacher. "My meditation is wonderful. I feel so aware, so peaceful, so alive. It's just delightful." The master once again said matter-of-factly, "It will pass."

This difficult lesson is amazing at helping with moodiness. When hardship comes, tell yourself, "This too shall pass," and even when life seems amazing, repeat, "This too shall pass." We should post signs of this wisdom everywhere to help all of us, children included, learn about the ephemerality of our emotions.

IS IT GOOD OR BAD? BEST NOT TO LABEL

The next strategy to explore in learning to move more quickly toward insight and problem-solving is to stop judging events as good or bad. Things happen; some changes are pleasant and some are not. Can you actually go through life without labeling what happens to you as good or bad? I am not saying bad things don't happen. Yes, they do, and bad things do happen to good people. But labeling them "bad" just makes it more difficult for you to be fluid. Somehow, you have to believe that even if a situation looks bad right now, in the grand scheme of things, there is good to be gleaned from it. I know, I know, UGH! I hate this lesson, but here goes. I used to say this to my kids all the time:

A young child, age three, sees a shiny object on the kitchen counter and wants it. He gets a chair and pushes it up to the counter to reach for the object.

His mother yells, "No! No!" and places the item where Johnny can't reach it.

But Johnny cries out, "I want it. I want it."

Johnny wanted a large knife. What appeared bad to Johnny (not getting the desired object) was really good for him. And what looked good to Johnny (the shiny object) was really bad for him. That's how we are supposed to view life. Hard, I know.

It's possible to decondition yourself from the habit of using these arbitrary categories. Instead of stopping to lament hard situations that *appear* to be dead ends, setbacks, or obstacles, accept them with the thought that this is the way it needs to be *right now*. Ancient Jewish wisdom teaches us that most difficult situations create opportunities for the most growth. But don't stop with acceptance. Instead, start looking for alternate routes.

I really like the work by Dr. Srikumar Rao, author of *Happiness at Work: Be Resilient, Motivated, and Successful—No Matter What*. In this book he writes, "Many who rise so triumphantly never label what they go through as bad and lament over it. They simply take it as a given as if they were a civil engineer surveying the landscape through which a road is to be built. In this view, a swamp is not a bad thing. It's merely something that has to be addressed in the construction plan." Dr. Rao goes on to say that the power of positive thinking may have helped some people; but for others, it just doesn't work. Those who can't see the good when difficulties occur become even more perturbed if they can't find a way out. He suggests paying close attention to your inner monologue and avoiding the words *good* and *bad* to describe what you are going though. Once you change your language, it will ultimately "leave you less vulnerable to life's sudden twists and turns."[10]

IT'S IMPORTANT TO recognize that the Cycle-of-Sanity exists because knowledge is power. When that next sense of frustration starts creeping up on you, don't label the situation as good or bad. Tell yourself, "This too shall pass," and then allow yourself to be flexible and fluid as you look forward to an "Aha" moment that brings such pleasure.

In the pages that follow, we will be exploring other tips and techniques that help make your moods easier to handle. Remember that each is natural and exists to teach you something important about yourself and your strengths. Don't get stuck in your moods, because that's where the trouble begins. Rather, learn to cycle through them.

CHAPTER THREE

CHARTING YOUR MOODS

Let's go back to the Cycle-of-Sanity. In Chapter 12, you'll find a blank Cycle-of-Sanity chart to help you follow your own progression as you move from frustration toward insight and happiness. Think of a situation you've been in that you were able to resolve—a fight with your husband, poor grades at school, an argument among your siblings, a social climber at the office. You'll write in what triggered your frustration, anger, and sadness. Then you'll track around to identify your "Aha" moment—the insight that came to you and gave you the energy to solve your problem. Use your own positive experience to remind yourself that you have the internal resources to help you get out of a negative mood and attain Moodtopia.

Once you've done this, you may think of other incidents. The more you reinforce your own capacity to resolve issues, the more confident you'll feel going forward. You can make several copies of the blank Cycle-of-Sanity chart and fill in your latest emotional ups and downs. Just to give you an example, here's how I would have charted my adventure with forty coats.

CREATE A MOODTOPIA CHART

Mood charting is an important step in getting in touch with your moodiness. When my clients use a Moodtopia chart, they begin to understand how and when their moods fluctuate. Instead of relying on your memory (which

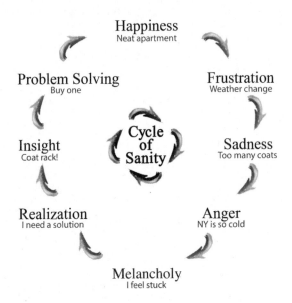

can be faulty), your Moodtopia chart will provide an objective record that you can ponder and analyze.

What is a mood chart? It's a place where you record in real time your fluctuating moods, hours of sleep, and mealtimes. These bodily functions are important. Living life in the fast lane, many women forget to eat, yet they haven't made the association between moodiness and low blood sugar. Others don't realize they're not sleeping enough.

In tracking your moods and detecting patterns in your moodiness, you will become more aware of the triggers that might previously have been invisible to you, and you'll be able to pinpoint when you feel at your best and worst. For instance, some of my clients discover that the time of day is important to how they feel. They chart feeling most down in the mornings, though others report that nighttime is worse for them.

The most effective way to chart your moods systematically is to find a good place to record them. There are many options for creating your own Moodtopia chart, depending on your personal preferences. If you're comfortable using Microsoft Word or Excel, you can devise a chart using spreadsheets—say, one per week. Something like the Daily Schedule in Chapter 12 would be a good start, since it has spaces for hourly entries. You could copy blank pages of this chart to track your moods and other issues week by week. Alternatively, you could buy a lovely, small journal to keep in your purse or a calendar to hang on the wall or take advantage of modern technology and use the daily calendar on your smartphone.

How should you use your Moodtopia chart? Jot down moments when you're feeling moody. Were there any triggers? Hunger, time of day, sleep patterns, or menstrual cycles should all be noted as well as interactions with others that set you off. You can simply list a few descriptive words or score your reactions on a scale of 1 to 10.

How long do you need to keep your Moodtopia chart? A month would be great, especially if you're a premenopausal woman, but even one week will open your eyes and make you more aware and in touch.

One of my instructors from homeopathy school, Dr. Joel Kreisberg, an integrative medicine physician and author of *Coaching and Healing: Transcending the Illness Narrative* suggests to his patients that they "track only one emotion at a time because following all of them becomes too daunting. For instance, you could note on your chart how often you feel frustration or sadness during one particular week."[1]

Tips for Making and Using Your Moodtopia Chart

Decide on the format you want to use.

Choose what you will be tracking. Mood charts can be as simple or elaborate as you make them. You may wish to follow one to two moods a week—or all of them. You can even track your exercise routine. It's totally up to you.

What to write down. You can simply list a few descriptive words or score your moods on a scale of 1 to 10.

Note anything significant that may have affected your mood. This could include: weather changes, sleeping partners, excess urination at night, an argument, hunger, alcohol, a cold, your menstrual cycle, a disturbing person or place. You are looking for patterns that can be personal triggers for you.

Determine how many times a day you would like to make entries in your chart. If you are awake for eighteen hours a day, it might be most helpful to chart three times a day—every six hours. Or you might make entries whenever your mood shifts.

Here's a brief example of how this may work for you:

My Moodtopia Chart					
Week: 1					
	Mon	**Tue**	**Wed**	**Thu**	**Fri**
6:00 AM					
6:30 AM			Kids woke me early. Didn't sleep well. Grr!		
7:00 AM	Woke up hungry	Crampy this morning. Ugh!			House is a mess. Distressing. No time to clean.
7:30 AM	Out of coffee! Bummer.		No one wants to eat the oatmeal I cooked.		
8:00 AM				Kids late for school this morning. Chaos!	
8:30 AM			Gotta get out of here. Ready to blow!		Morning went smoothly. Hurray!
9:00 AM	Boss likes my work. I'm pumped!	Low energy		Traffic getting to work. Late! Anxious.	
9:30 AM		My desk is a mess! Can't concentrate.			
10:00 AM	Jeremy gave me a hard time. Upset!			Can't get it together today. Feel down.	Jeremy wants to go out to dinner tonight.
10:30 AM			Happy to be at work		
11:00 AM		Coffee good!			Looking forward to our "date"
11:30 AM			Feeling tired and out of sorts.		
12:00 PM	Lunch with Kathy. Fun!	Feel like curling up in a ball!			Can't get a babysitter. Frantic!

Charting is not a test. Rather, it's simply a tool to help you become a more self-actualized person who is in greater control of your moods so they don't control you.

CREATE A MOODTOPIA JOURNAL

As an alternative or in addition to your Moodtopia chart, you may also want to keep a Moodtopia journal in which you write more expansively about your emotional ups and downs. If you've got the time, review each day's entries on your chart and then write a short summary in the evening to help you collect and think about what triggered your mood swings. Here's an example:

MOODTOPIA JOURNAL ENTRY
Tuesday, Jan. 25

I got grouchy at 1:30 because my meeting ran late and I hadn't eaten lunch yet—"hangry"! After I ate, I felt better and was more productive. But when I got home at 6 PM, I felt overwhelmed with kids' homework, making dinner, folding laundry. Fight over screen time. Exhausted. Went to bed tied in knots. Couldn't unwind. Had a hard time falling asleep. Upset that I yelled at the kids.

You might also consider copying the blank Cycle-of-Sanity graphic in Chapter 12 as a means to brainstorm. You could identify what was frustrating to you during the day . . . and then go around the cycle to come up with some solutions.

If you're really ambitious, you could create some questions that help you identify your emotional triggers. Try finishing these sentences in your Moodtopia journal. Just be aware that your answers may change with your life circumstances—so revisit this exercise from time to time:

1. The five things that make me frustrated are: _____
   _____

2. The five things that make me agitated are: _____
   _____

3. The five things that make me sad are: _____

_____

4. The five things that make me angry are: _____

_____

5. The five things that make me melancholy are: _____

_____

6. The people who upset me are: _____

_____

7. The places that feel unsafe to me are: _____

_____

You can use this information to explore your moods further in your Moodtopia journal as well as those successes you charted using the Cycle-of-Sanity graphic in Chapter 12.

PART II

Sara-Chana's Mood-Enhancing Herbs to the Rescue

CHAPTER FOUR

NOURISH YOUR LIVER AND REVITALIZE WITH ADAPTOGENS

Is life worth living? It all depends on the liver.

—WILLIAM JAMES

MILLIONS OF PEOPLE IN ALL CULTURES, FROM ALL SOCIOECONOMIC CLASSES, and all religions have used herbs continuously since the beginning of time. Healers throughout the ages have individualized herbal combinations for each person. They would look at the patient and prescribe a specific treatment and not necessarily just address a "diagnosis."

In 460 BC, Greek healer and physician Hippocrates used herbs as his platform for healing. He also recognized the significance of the mind-body connection. "It's more important to know what sort of person has a disease," he wrote, "than to know what sort of disease a person has." Like modern herbalists, he was more interested in understanding the personality of the patient and matching the herb to the individual than matching it to the ailment.

In the twelfth century, the famous Jewish doctor, philosopher, and scholar Maimonides recognized the connection between emotions and physical health. In *The Regimen of Health* (*De Regimine Sanitatis*), he discussed the link between mental and physical health, especially in relation to stress and anxiety, making him a pioneer in the development of psychosomatics. He formulated an herbal mix for stress and anxiety—a "stress-concoction"—that's still used today. And, many of the herbs it contains have been proven in modern clinical studies to reduce stress hormones. "This anti-anxiety," he wrote, "should be taken regularly, at all times. Its effects are that sadness and anxieties disappear. This is a remedy of which no equal can be found in gladdening, strengthening and invigorating the psyche. It should always be found in your possession."[1]

Despite this ancient knowledge, most people are still unaware of how their emotions affect their body. My instructor, integrative medicine physician Joel Kreisberg, taught us to not only look at what our clients were saying, but at which body parts were "falling apart." "From that," he said, "you will be able to better understand where their emotional health is standing. For instance," he continued, "if a person is complaining about heart disease, make sure to ask him, 'What broke your heart in your life?' Or, if she is complaining about losing her memory, ask her, 'What do you want to forget in your life?'"[2] The best way to cure the body is to cure the mind and its moods and emotions. A wonderful, safe way to do this is with herbs.

However, if you're new to herbal approaches to health and well-being, you may worry that an "alternative" treatment could easily be misused or could just be a waste of time and effort—and even money. But consider all the times you've sipped a cup of Sleepytime, Tension Tamer, or peppermint tea to unwind in the evening. Those are herbal remedies. Did you know that onions and garlic are considered herbs? Whenever you add these to your meals, you're ingesting botanicals. And your kitchen cabinet is filled with profoundly healing herbs and spices, such as ginger, curry, paprika, cinnamon, and turmeric.

Think about when you might have grabbed a packet labeled "Women's Remedy" at the drugstore checkout. That's another herbal preparation. Such over-the-counter products as these were formulated to help people the same way that pharmaceutical drugs do. And familiar medications you may have taken also come from plants. Digitalis is made from foxglove; quinine comes from the bark of the cinchona tree; aspirin is made from meadowsweet or white willow bark; and the product Glucophage, used in the treatment of diabetes, is derived from the herb goat's rue.

In Chapter 5, we will tackle mood-soothing herbs. But first, I want to recommend herbs that support the liver. The liver is your body's own detox organ—if you take care of your liver, it will take care of you! The liver-supporting herbs I recommend are known as cholagogues/choleretics. They stimulate the liver's production of bile and the secretion of bile from the gallbladder. They also have a laxative effect on the digestive system, since they increase the amount of bile in the duodenum.

In addition, I'll introduce you to herbs that support your nervous system so you can better deal with stress. These are called adaptogens. They calm your nerves so that your body learns new ways to cope. When your chemical reactions are more balanced, you will be better able to understand which mood herbs you require. You'll find a full explanation of the latter in the next chapter.

WHAT HAPPENS IN THE BRAIN WHEN YOU FEEL STRESSED?

You see a lion approaching (a danger you may not confront daily, but one that people certainly did face in the past) and neurochemical and electrical signals travel down your spinal cord to your two adrenal glands. These are no bigger than walnuts and each weighs less than a grape! They sit like tiny pyramids on top of your kidneys. Impulses from the brain tell them to release stress hormones, including adrenaline, which causes the uneasy sensation in your stomach and makes you feel panicky.[3] This increases the level of sugar in your blood, your heart rate, and your blood pressure—so you can run. Then, the hypothalamus signals the pituitary gland (at the base of the brain) to release factors that travel through the bloodstream to further stimulate the adrenals, which then produce the stress hormone cortisol. This gives you the strength to escape the approaching lion or other danger. Nowadays, it's what would enable a mother to lift a car if her child were beneath it.

Of course, the intensity of your reaction to extreme stress continues to be a vital survival tool. However, when you react as though a lion is about to attack if your train is delayed, or you miss an important work call, or you send the wrong text, your body won't function properly. It wasn't created to have these continuous emergency responses—only the occasional burst of stress hormones when you face real danger. Not all stress is bad. In fact, sometimes we crave it. But chronic stress is bad. If you're experiencing high stress responses daily, your liver will no longer function at its peak, your judgment can be skewed, and your adrenals can become overtaxed, making it difficult for you to be in control of your moods.

We actually crave it. Neuroendocrinologist, author, and professor Dr. Robert Sapolsky has written: "We all seek out stress. We hate the wrong kinds of stress, but when it's the right kind, we love it! We pay good money to be stressed by a scary movie, a roller coaster ride, a challenging puzzle."[4] There's also the phenomenon of "eustress"—the feeling of excitement when you're euphoric!

· ·

With chronic stress, these and other hormones may impact parts of the brain involved in memory formation, organization, and storage. Over time, this process can lead to confusion, memory loss, anger, and the inability to control your emotions. Indeed, studies at Yale University have shown that chronic stress reduces brain volume, leading to impaired cognition and emotional function. It can even cause your cells to age more quickly.[5]

Your liver stores and, when prompted by insulin, generates glucose—blood sugar.[6] But stress hormones will trigger the liver to produce *extra* blood sugar for that additional burst of energy at the moment of "perceived danger." This can cause the liver to be overtaxed and it may also leave you vulnerable for developing type 2 diabetes.[7] Depending on the long-term impact of whatever is bothering you—and how you handle it—after a big blowout, it could take anywhere from thirty minutes to a couple of days for your liver to return to its normal function.[8]

But the good news is that none of these changes have to be permanent. When your difficulties pass and you become calm again, your brain and body can rebound. Herbs can assist you in this process, so this is a very strong argument for using them.

WHY SUPPORT THE LIVER?

The word *liver* is rather aptly derived from the Old English word for "life." That makes perfect sense, as your liver is as indispensable as your heart or brain. Herbalists know that an optimally functioning liver increases vitality, vim, and vigor—and gives you a more serene life.

It can be difficult to diagnose when the liver is out of order because it's one organ that doesn't hurt when something is wrong with it. People can suffer for a long time from a liver ailment without realizing it. Herbalist Mary Bove, ND, author of *Herbs for Women's Health*, told me that one symptom of the liver being out of sync is waking in the wee hours of the morning. "Your liver may be crying out for support, especially if you often awaken around three a.m.," she said. According to Traditional Chinese Medicine (TCM), the liver rejuvenates and repairs itself between one and three a.m. Dr. Bove explained, "Often people who wake up around this time cannot fall back to sleep. This middle-of-the-night wakefulness can become a time for them to brood on their misery, thinking about all the wrongs that people have done to them, allowing dark and gloomy thoughts to dominate them, and they end up feeling unrefreshed when daylight appears."[9]

That's one of the reasons a liver that's congested and not functioning at its best can make you moody. I explain this concept to my clients this way: When you're drying clothes without having cleaned out the lint filter, your laundry will come out damp. But when the vent is cleaned, your clothes dry more efficiently. The same is true of your liver—as it's responsible for filtering your blood. It's the primary organ that breaks down and expels toxins from the body, so it needs to be in tip-top shape.

The famous herbalist Susun Weed, author of *Healing Wise*, has written, "Think of the liver as a recycling center. As the blood moves through the intricate network of cells that make up the liver, it is carefully examined. Metabolic by-products, hormones, cholesterol, vitamins, minerals, enzymes, bacteria, viral particles, and all the chemical detritus of living that are in the blood are judged: some are allowed to stay, others dismantled for recycling, and some tagged for removal."[10]

What About "Cleansing" or "Detoxifying" the Liver?

Your liver detoxes your body, but do you need to "detox" or "cleanse" the liver itself? Many powders, drinks, and pills in the marketplace claim to do just this. But are these claims valid? I don't think so. The herbalist philosophy is: We don't need to detox! Instead, we need to support and nourish the liver and gallbladder so they work at their peak. The liver doesn't need cleaning because this amazing organ cleans itself! Herbalist David Winston, author of *Adaptogens: Herbs for Strength, Stamina, and Stress Relief,* explained to me why he wasn't a fan of "cleansing protocols." "Our bodies are inherently self-cleaning," he told me. "They're capable of regularly eliminating metabolic wastes via the liver, bowel, kidneys, skin, and lungs to maintain our health."[11]

. . . . ⁖ . . . .

Your liver also plays an important role in the digestion of proteins, sugar, and fat. Herbalist Amanda McQuade Crawford, author of *Herbal Remedies for Women,* told me, "Herbalists understand the body to be *self-*regulating, with an in-built design for self-healing and self-cleansing. The liver is one of the miraculous ways our bodies filter out 'problem' compounds, including many germs, to protect us." This is particularly true for women. Our bodies require more fat than men's. But this fat, according to Crawford, is "vulnerable to the increased number of toxins we're all exposed to in our modern environment. The liver detoxifies many of these toxins that can build up in the fat stored by women. That's why supporting the liver is so important."[12]

The gallbladder is the liver's partner in keeping us healthy. During an interview, herbalist David Winston explained the role of gallbladder health in relation to your liver. "The liver also secretes a fat-digesting fluid known as bile, some of which is stored in the gallbladder," he told me. "Bile is our body's natural laxative and the liver dumps wastes filtered from the bloodstream into the bile for excretion via the bowel." Sometimes and for various reasons, the liver doesn't produce enough bile. This can cause constipation, clay-colored stools, impaired fat digestion, and gasiness. "Many herbs known as choleretics/cholagogues stimulate bile secretion from the liver or bile excretion from the gallbladder. These bitter-tasting herbs include gentian root, dandelion root, artichoke leaf . . ."[13] (I will discuss them in greater detail later in this chapter.)

Guido Masé, my Italian herbalist friend and author of the book *The Wild Medicine Solution: Healing with Aromatic, Bitter, and Tonic Plants,*[14] told me during a recent interview, "In Italian, anger is called *collera,* which has been translated to mean 'too much bile backed up into your system.' It was taught in Italy that the way to reduce anger and irritability was to stimulate the liver to release bile. So, for generations, angry people were encouraged to eat more bitter foods and use bitter herbs to dispel and pass their anger."[15]

······· Eat Your Bitters! ·····································

Many traditional cultures believe it's important that all five flavors—salty, spicy, sour, sweet, and bitter—are represented in the diet. Each flavor has a specific effect on the body. Guido Masé told me, "As human beings, we evolved consuming a diversified diet. At the beginning of the twentieth century, 80 percent of our calories came from 120 plant species, most of which were rich in the bitterness. (Today, that same 80 percent comes from six to ten different plants.)"[16] But with the birth of industrial agriculture and food processing, the bitterness was stripped away in exchange for mostly pleasant flavors—sweet and salty. Most modern diets have tons of salty, spicy, sour, and sweet flavors, but are devoid of bitterness, which is associated with the digestive system and liver function.

Herbalists recommend eating bitter foods that help support digestion and stimulate the liver to work at its optimal level. So, include more bitter plants and greens in your diet. Try radicchio, dandelion greens, rapini, endive, kale, daikon, arugula, dill, horseradish, watercress, parsley, radish, cilantro, fenugreek seeds, basil, mustard greens, and romaine lettuce.

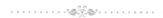

Besides, living in our modern world, it makes sense that our liver is stressed and needs support, as every day we absorb a frightful potpourri of *xenobiotics*—foreign chemicals in the body coming from the environment, medications, or pollutants. These include such contaminants as pesticides sprayed on fruits and vegetables, phthalates in plastics and cosmetics, chlorine in household cleaners, and PCBs and heavy metals in farm-raised fish, to name just a few. Being the largest solid organ, the liver can also be adversely affected by poor diet, certain lifestyle choices (such as staying up all night, watching too much TV, or spending too much time on your smartphone), alcohol consumption, and taking acetaminophen or other nonprescription painkillers.

External and emotional stressors, such as long lines at the supermarket, work aggravations, parking tickets, crashing computers, drastic weight-loss diets, confusing relationships, divorce, parenting challenges, family illnesses, lack of sleep, anxiety, and exploding anger can also impede the liver's function.

Why is this so? When your body is in a stressed state, you operate within your sympathetic nervous system (the part that accelerates heart rate, constricts blood vessels and digestion, and raises blood pressure to prepare you for an emergency). When the body is dominated by this system, it diverts resources to the muscles (fight or flight) and away from organs (rest and digest). Our current lifestyle promotes the sympathetic nervous system to be turned on far too often. If you wake up feeling nauseated, this indicates that your liver is having a hard time. Tense muscles signify that energy is being shunted away from your repair and renewal system—and that means your liver will not be detoxifying your blood optimally. This is why your liver needs assistance—to stay strong and work to its fullest capacities.

A liver that needs support manifests in the body as physical symptoms, such as rashes and constipation. When choosing which herb is best for you, herbalists will evaluate the symptoms of a congested liver. Ask yourself a few questions:

- When I am stressed, do I get constipated or have loose stools?
- Do I get skin rashes?
- Do I feel extremely sluggish?
- Do I lose my appetite?
- Do I drink too much alcohol?
- Do I awaken in the middle of the night and have trouble falling asleep again?

Indeed, moodiness can result if your liver isn't functioning at its best. Since you're taking a global approach to controlling your emotions so they don't control you, having a highly functioning liver will give you the strength you need to achieve your goals. Even if you make correct lifestyle choices, just living in today's stressful world will cause your liver to need more support. But if you've lived a life filled with unhealthful foods, too much alcohol, and lots of anger, then including one of the following herbs will be essential in revitalizing your liver and improving your well-being.

HERBS THAT SUPPORT THE LIVER

When you are selecting herbs to support your liver, gravitate to the ones that most closely match your life situation. If you're purchasing these products, you'll often find that companies make a blend of herbs. That's totally fine. These are called liver supports, liver tonics, or "bitters." Whichever formulation you buy, make sure to pick one that says on the label "liver support" and *not* "cleanse" or "detox." I suggest to my clients that they take herbs in tincture or liquid form rather than capsules, because they're absorbed better that way. (Please see Chapter 5 for information on how these are prepared.) Dosage depends on your weight. Typically for adults, I recommend 25 to 45 drops two to three times a day—before meals if possible. As recommended earlier, check with your registered herbalist or health-care provider about any contraindications before beginning a course of liver-support herbs.

Most of the following herbs are known as bitters. You will see a difference after thirty days. How long should you take the herb before you eat? Just five to ten minutes. But even if taken in middle of meal, you can gain benefit.

Artichoke Leaves (*Cynara scolymus*)

Artichoke leaves help regenerate the liver because they stimulate the flow of bile from the liver to the gallbladder, where toxins can be removed. This can help with digestion.

Indication: This is my favorite herb choice for anyone who struggles with indigestion. Often, if the liver is unable to properly break down the fats in foods, people can struggle with GERD (gastroesophageal reflux disease). Although this plant alone will not cure GERD, the reflux of food is an indication that it is needed.

Burdock Root (*Arctium lappa*)

Burdock root is edible. Worldwide, people mix it into stir-fries and soups. It's a tasty addition to your diet, but it's also an excellent liver support. This herb also aids with skin conditions, including eczema, psoriasis, acne, and dermatitis. These ailments often manifest when the liver is overloaded with a diet high in fat and protein that the body can't break down.

Indication: I suggest this herb when my clients not only complain of moodiness but also about their troubling skin. It may be dry, oily skin, or easily damaged, or wounds may take longer to heal.

Culver Root (*Veronicastrum virginicum*)

Culver root is a powerful liver support. Only a small amount is needed. It can assist the liver and gallbladder by increasing the production and secretion of bile, which lubricates the intestines. This, in turn, enhances bowel movements.

Indication: I suggest this herb when my client's system has been under a lot of stress. Improper diet and stress may affect the bowels, creating bloating, constipation, diarrhea or hemorrhoids.

Dandelion Root (*Taraxacum officinale*)

This is the root of the common dandelion plant—yes, the one you're always trying to yank out of your lawn. Hidden beneath the green leafy plant with the wonderful highlighter-yellow flowers is the root—the part that helps nourish the liver. Dandelion root has been celebrated as a liver support throughout the ages because it stimulates bile flow. Herbalists often use it to help fight fatty liver, cirrhosis, estrogen dominance, and also acne.

Indication: I suggest this plant for clients whose legs or feet tend to swell. It also helps people who don't urinate as often as they should.

Gentian Root (*Gentiana lutea*)

Gentian root is used specifically to protect the liver, stimulate its function, help cell proliferation, and increase the flow of bile. It is also known to inhibit the development of viruses that affect the liver. According to the University of Maryland Medical Center, gentian is often used in Europe to treat anemia by stimulating the digestive system to more easily absorb iron and other nutrients.[17]

Indication: I suggest this for clients who suffer from such digestive problems as GERD, or who feel sluggish after they eat, and also to clients prone to anemia.

Milk Thistle Seed (*Silybum marianum*)

Milk thistle has been used across the globe for generations due to its remarkable effects on the liver and gallbladder. It helps with the detoxification of poisons (such as alcohol), can help regenerate damaged liver tissue, stimulates bile production, and improves digestion. It is rare that I suggest herbs in capsule form, but this is one herb that performs well in that modality. The customary use was to grind the seeds and add them to porridge. Today, I recommend four capsules before breakfast and dinner.

Indication: I suggest this herb to anyone who has been on a medication for a long time—especially women coming off long-term use of birth control pills or pain medications. It's also helpful for people who have seasonal allergies or catch colds or flu frequently. Milk thistle is not recommended for use with birth control pills because it can undermine their effectiveness.

Watercress (*Nasturtium officinale*)

Watercress is a food and an herb. It's a tasty but bitter green in the cruciferous family, so it's related to cabbage, arugula, cauliflower, and broccoli. It's rich in phytochemicals called glucosinolates that contain sulfur. This compound enhances your liver's filtering abilities, has a cooling effect on the body, and aids digestion. Hippocrates described it as a stimulant and expectorant.

Indication: This herb complements other herbs in a blend. You can also add it to a salad mix as a great way to sneak in bitters.

Yellow Dock Root (*Rumex crispus*)

Yellow dock root is known as a blood purifier and is commonly used to remove toxins. It helps break down fatty foods by stimulating bile production, enhancing normal liver detoxification and improving the flow of digestive juices. It also has mild diuretic effects, which help flush harmful substances. It can reduce irritation of the liver and digestive system.

Indication: I choose this herb for clients who are anemic or feel sluggish, who have had a long illness, and who have trouble eating enough protein. Yellow dock has a lot of natural iron and is easily absorbed.

ADAPTOGENS

After you've begun your liver-support routine, the next step in preparing your body is to start taking an adaptogen. I recommend these as overall wellness tonics. Using a "tonic" to restore balance and health is an ancient idea. As David Winston explained, "'Adaptogen' is a relatively new way of describing a type of remedy commonly found in traditional Chinese (Qi tonic), African (Manyasi), Tibetan, Ayurvedic (Rasayana), and Cherokee medicine."[18] These agents don't alter the mind; rather, they help the entire body function optimally during times of stress. In fact, they bring your body back from an extreme to a balanced state. They're called adaptogens because of their unique ability to *adapt* their function to your body's specific needs. As a consequence, they literally help you adapt to your environment, allowing you to better handle stress, whether mental or physical.

Adaptogens work slowly and subtly, but over time they strengthen your body's response to stress and enhance your ability to cope with anxiety and fatigue. But patience is important—you have to give them time to undo all the stress that has accumulated in the body. (Think of the tortoise and the hare.)

As I explained earlier, in modern society our body is constantly in a state of stress. Our system was created for the fight-or-flight response—we see a lion and we run. But people who live in today's cities remain in this mode most of the time. Because of the pervasive impact of urban life, we're always stressed—adrenaline at the ready. And that can make us moody!

Your adrenal glands are important for your overall health and should be in perfect balance to help you stay in charge of your emotions. They produce vital hormones, including cortisol, that work in conjunction with adrenaline and noradrenaline to regulate your reactions to stress. Adaptogens are a unique group of herbs that address your chronic and acutely stressful moments by improving the health of your adrenal system. Introducing adaptogens into your daily routine will help you reduce the damage that the adrenal system can produce when you are under stress.

. . . . **What About Adrenal Burnout?** . . . .

Just like the buzzwords *liver detox*, the term *adrenal burnout* seems all the rage these days. But is this a bona fide syndrome and must it be addressed? Master herbalist and teacher David Winston told me, "There is adrenal insufficiency, which is rare and causes serious disease. But there is no such thing as 'adrenal burnout.' I think people are really describing the negative effects of chronic stress, with elevated cortisol levels and HPA axis or SAS dysfunction. And yes, herbs can help this—especially adaptogens and nervines."[19]

. . . . ⚜ . . . .

Most of the research on adaptogens has occurred with athletes in China and Russia, where these herbs are used to maintain competitors' health and enhance their performance.[20] Researchers find that they can put these athletes into abnormally difficult situations both physically and emotionally. But when they use adaptogens, the athletes recover faster and maintain their health.

Adaptogens work well with your liver-support herbs and they blend even more beautifully with the mood herbs discussed in Chapter 5. At some point, you'll find the perfect combination of liver support, adaptogens, and mood herbs. You'll take them two to three times a day to help your life run more smoothly. For now, simply choose one to three adaptogens from the following list or a blend from a reputable company that most closely matches your life situation. The dosage for all of them is 25 to 40 drops diluted in juice or water two to three times a day. These herbs can be taken with or without food. I use them in tincture form. Just note that ginsengs can be quite stimulating, so begin with small doses and find what works best for you. Rhodiola has a slight stimulating effect which is less intense than ginseng if you find the latter is too much for you.

American Ginseng Root (*Panax quinquefolius*)

The genus *Panax* comes from the Greek word *panacea*, meaning "all healing." American ginseng is mildly stimulating. It's known for its ability to fight physical and mental fatigue. It helps a person find energy that may be hidden in his or her body. It is also used for chronic stress with depression or anxiety. It can mitigate burnout, compromised immune systems, and insomnia. Athletes throughout the world use this herb while training, to boost their strength and stamina. Students often take it while studying because it helps them maintain a high level of mental alertness and improves memory.

Indications: I suggest this herb to clients who feel they need a gentle push to get through their day. They may have slightly high cholesterol, feel sluggish midday, and have a cloudy mind. It's considered a "cooling" ginseng and is best for people who tend to feel hot or who get heated when they become angry or moody.

Ashwagandha Root (*Withania somnifera*)

Ashwagandha has been part of Ayurvedic medicine for generations. This herb calms the system and has traditionally been used for anxiety, bad dreams, mild obsessive-compulsive disorder (OCD), insomnia, and nervous exhaustion. It simultaneously stimulates and calms the central nervous system, creating a balance. It also lowers cortisol levels, which reduces the feeling of stress in the body.

Indications: I suggest this herb when a person has worked too hard without taking a break. It also can assist the body if you've been through an illness or catch cold too easily. Ashwagandha can gently stimulate thyroid function, and many people who are borderline hypothyroid benefit from it. This herb also increases libido.

Asian Ginseng Root (*Panax ginseng*)

Red ginseng is the most stimulating of the adaptogens; it increases capillary circulation in the brain. It is useful for people who lack energy and feel "played out" or overtired. Traditionally, it has been used for depression, exhaustion, and insomnia. Since this herb gives a wonderful "push" to the system, I recommend refraining from taking it after six p.m.

Indications: I suggest this ginseng to clients who are exhausted and can't muster the energy to get through their day. This herb is powerful and gives one energy to perform better and remain alert. It does not work like caffeine and does not give that feeling of coming off an adrenaline rush. I recommend it to clients who describe themselves as having "brain fog."

Cordyceps Fungus (*Cordyceps sinensis*)

Cordyceps is a wonderfully versatile medicinal mushroom that has many applications. In fact, doctors in China have used it for more than two thousand years. The risk of cognitive decline and dementia increases with age, but research suggests that cordyceps helps keep the brain healthy with age, both structurally and functionally. Cordyceps is believed to enhance athletic performance.

Indications: I recommend cordyceps to clients who have worked too hard and not taken enough time for themselves. It's used for chronic stress, fatigue, tendency to catch colds and flu easily, and also for extreme athletic training. It also improves libido.

Eleuthero Root or Siberian Ginseng (*Eleutherococcus senticosus*)

Eleuthero works to balance such brain chemicals as serotonin, norepinephrine, dopamine, and epinephrine. Its effect on these mood-determining brain chemicals makes it a natural mood stabilizer. Germany's Commission E approved Siberian ginseng as a tonic in times of fatigue and debility, declining capacity for work or concentration, and during convalescence. (You'll learn more about Commission E on page 58.) It can improve athletic performance and increase muscle strength. When taken regularly, it enhances immune function, reduces cortisol (stress), and helps improve cognitive and physical performance.

Indications: I recommend eleuthero to clients who have burned the candle on both ends. They are overstressed, undernourished but overfed, don't get enough sleep or exercise, and/or have dark circles under their eyes.

Holy Basil, a.k.a. Tulsi (*Ocimum tenuiflorum, O. sanctum Sanskrit, O. gratissumum*)

Holy basil is known in India as the "elixir of anti-aging." It is a gentle plant in the mint family. This herb has been purported to benefit the mind, body, and soul for generations. It is believed that holy basil decreases stress hormones.

Indications: I suggest holy basil for mild depression and sadness. It's slow-acting but can help women fight fatigue and stress; boost their immune system; and regulate blood sugar, blood pressure, and hormone levels so people feel more balanced.

Rhodiola Root (*Rhodiola rosea*)

Rhodiola is a mild stimulant that enhances memory and improves mild depression, impaired cognitive function, exhaustion, and weakness. It's also used as an immune tonic. It's believed that rhodiola increases the body's tolerance to stress by influencing key brain chemicals, such as serotonin, norepinephrine, and beta-endorphins. It is said to bolster the healing properties of one's own nervous system. It's slow-working, but the healing is deep and long-lasting.

Indications: I suggest this herb for people who are burned out, feel as if they lack energy, or are slightly depressed. It can reduce mental and physical fatigue and increase the body's energy. However, those who are anxious, manic, or have bipolar disorder should avoid using it.

Schisandra Berries/Seeds (*Schisandra chinensis*)

The schisandra berry is called the "five-flavor fruit": It is sweet, sour, salty, bitter, and pungent all at once. You don't eat this berry, but it's used medicinally. It's mildly stimulating and at the same time produces a calm, focused state of mind. It's used to retard aging, increase energy, fight fatigue, and improve sexuality. It counters stress by reducing the levels of cortisol in the blood. It also sharpens concentration, decreases mental fatigue, and increases accuracy and quality of work. It can enhance your capacity for physical and mental stress. It also improves resistance to disease, energy, physical performance, and endurance.

Schisandra is also popular among woman for its ability to make the skin soft, smooth, and beautiful. It has been taken for hundreds of years in China for this purpose. It is believed to work by balancing the fluids of the skin.[21]

Indications: I suggest this herb to women who feel balanced but want to improve their overall health and well-being. It helps the body gently balance itself. Berries are good for our body, and this healing berry is tops on my list. It's not strong, but it's subtly powerful.

WHEN YOU BEGIN a program of liver support and adaptogens, you will prepare your body for the main course—the herbs I recommend for reaching Moodtopia. You'll find all of these in the following chapter. So, just jump in!

CHAPTER FIVE

MOOD HERBS TO THE RESCUE

> The art of healing comes from nature and not from the physician. Therefore, the physician must start from nature with an open mind.
>
> —PARACELSUS

THERE'S LITTLE VALUE TO YOURSELF OR YOUR FAMILY IN STOICALLY "KEEP-ing it together" and "trying your best," when it's obvious that you're on an emotional rollercoaster. At these moments, you need tools to help you cope, and that's where botanical medicine comes in. As the healers of old knew, if you allow yourself to remain in negative states for too long, your physical health will eventually be compromised. And no one needs to spiral down that path.

That's where herbs come in. They help build your emotional immune system. They calm and center. They heal shattered and frazzled nerves. They help you appreciate life's joys. Herbs move you along the road to see clearly what you must do to heal yourself. You can safely use them *before* desperation sets in. When you combine self-awareness and daily self-care with herbal remedies customized to your moods, personality, and needs, you actually take yourself off the scary emotional ride.

In this chapter, I'll walk you through the hows and whys of herbs so you can develop your own herbal remedy plan for everyday and special times. I delineate which are most calming, which are most helpful in alleviating stress, and which are especially useful for handling hormonal cycles that can throw off the most even-tempered woman. These tools are a gift you can give yourself and that I give to my clients.

HOW TO BEGIN: USING HERBS SAFELY, GENTLY, AND WITH EXPERTISE

Today, many doctors, herbalists, and pharmacists rely on the German Commission E for its thorough research on herbs and their actions. This institution has compiled data on the most commonly used herbs. The Monographs, primarily published by the German Commission E between 1983 and 1993, are an authoritative description of the uses and side effects of more than three hundred herbs and herbal combinations (known as *phyto-medicines*, literally "plant medicines"). They are based on strict scientific investigation, and to ensure objectivity, the work of the Commission E was entirely financed by the German government. The Monographs are recognized globally and are used by herbalists, pharmacies, and medical doctors alike.

In addition, other scientific studies are becoming available from around the world daily. In the United States, you can locate summaries of the latest research from the National Center for Complementary and Integrative Health (NCCIH) which is part of the US Department of Health and Human Services. This office has a section on its website called "Herbs at a Glance" where you'll find descriptions of plants and their actions (see (https://nccih.nih.gov/health/herbsataglance.htm).[1]

Many people fear that the manufacture and sale of herbal medicines aren't regulated by the US Food and Drug Administration (FDA). However, this fear is unfounded. The FDA's comprehensive regulations govern the handling and processing of herbs, testing requirements, record keeping procedures, labeling, and advertising, among other activities. The manufacturing sites of companies I suggest are inspected by FDA officials to ensure their rules are followed and that the herbal products they produce are safe. As time progresses, more and more double-blinded research studies are being conducted on herbs and their effects on our mind and body. Most herbalists have studied extensively in their field and also rely heavily on the writings of the ancient herbal healers from both the West and East. What we're finding is that most of the research studies confirm what has long been known about the positive effects of herbal medicine on the human body.

Nevertheless, the number of double-blinded clinical research investigations of herbal remedies is tiny compared to what exists in the pharmaceutical world. My teacher, David Winston, explains why: "Medical and drug research in the US is usually sponsored by drug companies," he told me. "For the most part, this research is extremely expensive and few herb companies have the resources to fund such research. It is also difficult, if not impossible, to patent herbal products so there's little incentive for pharmaceutical companies to study them as they are unlikely to recoup their investments. So, the number of clinical trials using herbs in this country is quite small."[2]

On the other hand, governments of many other countries fund this kind of research. Clinical trials to explore the efficacy of herbal medicine in human disease in China, India, Japan, South Korea, Taiwan, and Iran are ongoing. In addition, in France, Germany, Italy, and Sweden several large phytopharmaceutical companies are conducting their own research on herbal products and running clinical trials.

SOME PRACTICAL MATTERS

Before you dive in, here are some of the most common questions about how to obtain and use herbs.

Do I Need to Work with an Herbalist?
What If I Can't Find One in My Community?

It's best to start your herbal journey with a master herbalist. In this book, I discuss each herb separately so you can get a feel for the action each may have on your emotions. However, I recommend relying on experts. The herbs can be taken separately or they may be combined to meet your specific needs because, as you know, you can feel anxious and sad and agitated and unsexual all at the same time! As the great herbalist Donald Yance said, "Herbalists most often use a combination of herb formulas and not just single herbs—they think of the herbs as harmonizing each other and working together like a great jazz band."[3] Professionals usually combine three to seven herbs. Herbalist David Winston explains why: "We are treating complex people with complex problems and to do that you often need complex formulas."[4] When you work with an herbalist, he or she will listen closely to what you're saying and create a formula that works for the specific challenges you're facing.

· · · · · · · · · **Seven Combinations You Can Safely Try** · · · · · · · · · · · · · · · ·

Anxiety/stress: bacopa, fresh milky oats, skullcap

Sadness/the blues: holy basil, mimosa bark, motherwort, Saint-John's-wort

Grumpy/short fuse: chamomile, valerian, motherwort, skullcap

Brain fog: eleuthero, rosemary, schisandra, bacopa

Burnout/exhaustion: rhodiola, fresh milky oats, ashwagandha

Insomnia: California poppy, lemon balm, linden, passion flower

Lack of libido: damiana, ashwagandha, rose, mimosa

· · · · · · · · · · · ❧ · · · · · · · · · · · ·

That means most herbalists will spend from one to three hours taking a proper history. You may discuss your childhood, challenging illnesses, nutrition, medications, exercise regimens, and family history, to name a few. The more professionals understand your strengths and weaknesses and your lifestyle choices, the better able they'll be to choose the best botanicals for your body type, personality, and medical issues. They'll work diligently to find a program that you can easily comply with.

Most people can safely take just about all of the herbs I've listed here. You can experiment with them as long as you take the proper dosage (see pages 61–62). But if you feel uncomfortable doing this on your own, you can find an herbalist in your area by searching the American Herbalists Guild's (AHG) website: www.americanherbalistsguild.com. AHG herbalists each have a minimum of ten years' experience and have worked with more than one thousand clients to qualify. They must also pass a series of exams before being accepted into the guild. Most AHG herbalists are familiar with diseases as well as pharmaceuticals and their interactions with herbs. An AHG herbalist can help you decide which are best for your issues.

If no master herbalist is available, with care and patience it's possible to find a single herb or create your own combination to help balance yourself. When you understand the individual properties of the herbs, you can formulate your own blend targeted to your needs, especially if you're already experienced with herbal treatments. In that case, you may already have a few go-to remedies that have worked for you in the past.

Where Can I Find These Herbs? Are There Any Brands You Recommend?

You can grow medicinal herbs in your garden or on a windowsill. You can also purchase them in bulk from many reputable companies. You would make them either into a tea or, for a stronger dose, into an infusion. Herbs in these forms are extremely beneficial but, in industrialized countries, and for those unfamiliar with growing herbs, I suggest purchasing them at a local health food store or online.

My favorite companies for trustworthy, safe herbals and tinctures are: Herbalist and Alchemist, Herb Pharm, Herbs Etc., Herbs of Light, Standard Process, Mountain Rose Herbs, Healing Spirit Farm, Woodland Essence, WishGarden Herbs, Frontier Co-op, Urban Moonshine, Gaia, and Eclectic Herbs (see Resources for contact information). Additional reliable companies are popping up every day. Just call to make sure that a qualified herbalist is overseeing their ingredient purchases.

How Do I Take the Herbs?

Although herbs are sold in pill or capsule form, I've found that with a few exceptions, tinctures are the way to go. A tincture is the liquid by-product of a plant that has steeped in grain alcohol or glycerite for six to eight weeks to extract its healing properties. Tinctures are portable and easy to use.

If you're not working with a master herbalist, it's best to buy already prepared tinctures. If you are working with an herbalist, the process begins when your herbalist properly identifies the plant(s) to be used. The root, leaves, stems, flowers, seeds, or the whole plant can be utilized. The herbalist may include all of the components or only a few. Herbalists usually prefer fresh plants, but certain herbs used in tinctures are better if they're dried. After six to eight weeks, the liquid is strained and the wilted material is discarded, leaving only the tincture behind. When it's ready, it's properly labeled and placed in a dark glass bottle with a glass dropper.

What Dosage Should I Take? How Can I Determine That for Myself?

The typical adult dose is 25 drops of tincture diluted in a shot glass (1 ounce) of water or juice, two to three times a day. Some people require more drops (45 to 65), whereas others need only a few to feel the herbs' effects. If you're uncertain how much to take, begin with a few drops and increase until you feel less anxious, reactive, or moody. The typical dose is two to three times daily unless directed otherwise by your herbalist or health-care professional.

Whether or not one works with a master herbalist, most people feel the calming effects within twenty minutes of taking the preparation. But to get the full, long-term effects, it's best to continue regular use for three to six weeks. I usually tell my clients to come in for a follow-up in six weeks. That's when we'll have a better assessment of the herbs' effectiveness.

Children's Dosages

Reducing the adult dose of an herb down to a pediatric "serving size" doesn't guarantee an accurate dose for a child. When the adult dose is 2 dropperfuls (60 drops), the following is recommended for children. Remember always to dilute the herb in a little juice or a sweet drink:

Age	Dosage
Younger than 3 months	2 drops
3 to 6 months	3 drops
6 to 9 months	4 drops
9 to 12 months	5 drops
12 to 18 months	7 drops
18 to 24 months	8 drops
2 to 3 years	10 drops
3 to 4 years	12 drops
4 to 6 years	15 drops[5]

Some extracts are unsuitable for children. Consult your herbalist for advice. As with your own health, be sure to consult your child's health-care practitioner for any contraindications.

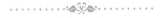

MOODTOPIA HERBS

Now that you've been introduced to the world of botanicals, let's look at how some specific herbs have helped my patients regulate their moods and how they can help you. Most (but not all) of the herbs below are in a category called *nervines*. They support and nourish the nervous system. They are used to relieve nagging muscle tension and spasms, circular thoughts, insomnia, fear, anxiety, and anger. When taken regularly, they not only help relax the physical body, but also restore and support healthy nerve function. I will also discuss their anti-depressant, sedative, anti-anxiety (anxiolytic), and adaptogenic properties.

I've listed them alphabetically for easy reference.

> **Bacopa (*Brahmi monnier*)** This is a traditional Ayurvedic (Indian) medicinal used to regain energy and focus, eliminate brain fog, and for mood regulation. This herb is an adaptogen and also anxiolytic (antianxiety agent). According to the University of Michigan Health System, it supports the effects of certain neurotransmitters including serotonin and acetylcholine.

Recently retired, Olivia was apprehensive about the life she was about to create now that she had a lot of free time. She found herself staying in bed too long. Although she was catching up on her reading, she admitted that she was getting anxious about her future. Olivia still had energy, but she was unsure how to use it. She also felt her eyesight was getting weaker and had been to an eye doctor who said this was due to aging.

Bacopa is known to help a person who begins to feel visual weakness, so this herb instantly popped into my mind as she spoke to me. It's also a nerve tonic and is purported to enhance vitality and longevity. Olivia was far too young and had way too much spunk to abandon productivity, so I felt she would love this herb. We spent the next hour discussing charity work she could do and her eyes lit up. Her previous life had been so busy—working, raising her children, and keeping her house in order—she never had time to be bored, and she had few opportunities for charity work. "What a brilliant idea!" she said. I suggested she take bacopa three times a day and get back to me in a month.

At our next visit, Olivia said with glee, "I'm shocked to admit that my eyesight seems clearer and sharper. And guess what else? I'm cooking two mornings a week at a homeless shelter, I'm reading books to children at our local library, I joined my church choir (they accepted me even though I don't have a great voice), I'm working out once a week with a trainer, and I'm taking a pottery class. By the way, I don't have time to be anxious. It doesn't fit into my busy schedule." I will admit that my genius suggestions helped create a new and exciting life for Olivia, and okay, we can also give a little credit to the wonderful herb bacopa!

> **Blue vervain (*Verbena hastata*)** This antianxiety herb works on the parasympathetic nervous system and is commonly used for panic attacks, nervous tension, insomnia, anxiety, irritability, and lethargy. A mood booster that helps with depression, it's often used as a restorative and recuperative herb.

Jackie lectured about education to teachers, school boards, and parents. She was self-confident, assured, and articulate. She had been my client earlier for various issues, but called me frantically one morning. "I don't know what happened," she cried. "When I woke up this morning, I had what I think is another panic attack!" She said that for the last two weeks, out of the blue, she would suddenly get panicky, break into a cold sweat, and feel nausea. She was on her way to a speaking engagement when she called me and decided to take a cab rather than the train, fearing she wouldn't be able to tolerate crowds. She passed on coffee, afraid the caffeine would agitate her further. Somehow she made it through her speech.

Later, she called me back, and I suggested she visit her doctor to be sure there was no physical cause for her symptoms. She made an appointment with me for the following morning. When she arrived, she was obviously shaken. She had a stressful life, but she'd never panicked! We spent the next two hours talking about ways to find calmness. We reviewed eating, sleeping, exercising—the usual. She realized she wasn't taking care of herself and was trying to save the world at her own expense. I reminded her of the well-known example: you need to put on your own oxygen mask before helping others on the plane. She laughed and agreed. But just because she understood what was going on, didn't mean her body would recover immediately.

I suggested to Jackie that she begin taking the herb blue vervain three times a day to take the edge off, while she worked on changing her lifestyle. As she began managing her panic and making some changes in her life, she reduced the dosage to twice a day and then once a day. She weaned off it after a couple of months and only used it when she felt the panic coming on again.

Blue vervain is one of my favorite herbs for panic—which Jackie will attest to. It's needed in acute cases, but once my client works out where the panic is coming from, the blue vervain finds a special place in the cabinet and she has confidence knowing it's there when she needs it.

> **California poppy (*Eschscholzia californica*)** This sedative herb is a member of the poppy family and somewhat distantly related to the opium poppy. It's used specifically to relieve insomnia but also soothes anxiety and nervous tension.

Adriane was a workaholic and loved it. The CEO of a large company, she was always juggling twenty tasks at once while traveling the world. She was smart, savvy, and capable. She'd been my client earlier for chronic sinus infections after her endless rounds of antibiotics failed to clear them. She felt as a successful businesswoman, it was improper for her to always have a tissue in her hand, so she sought other options—and my interventions did the trick.

But one day, Adriane called me from Europe in despair. She couldn't fall asleep anymore. In fact, she hadn't slept for four nights in a row. A visit to the local doctor landed her with a prescription for sleeping pills. They made her so groggy the next morning, she felt sleepless nights were a more viable choice. She made an appointment to see me straightaway when she landed. We reviewed what was going on in her life. She confided that she'd planned to marry the man she was dating, but out of nowhere (or at least she missed it), he'd called off the wedding. Embarrassed, heartbroken, and bewildered, she didn't know what to do and would lay in bed for hours tossing and turning.

As an herbalist, I couldn't solve the problem with her now-ex, but we did speak about learning to breathe deeply and visualize what she wanted in a future husband. We also discussed her former fiancé and examined why the relationship didn't work. But, alas, I am not a psychologist. I am an herbalist, and so I turned to my herbs for help. Adriane was the perfect candidate for California poppy. I advised her that she shouldn't take herbs to assist with sleep right before bedtime. She was to begin about three hours before she turned in, and then again an hour before. They get into the system slowly. Well, Adriane found a new friend in California poppy. It took a good two weeks for her to get back into a normal sleep pattern, but California poppy became a staple, right next to her sinus herbs.

Chamomile (*Matricaria recutita, Chamaemelum nobile*) This nervine herb is extraordinarily gentle, subtle, and effective in calming anxiety and stress. It's also helpful for panic attacks, muscle twitches, and insomnia. Chamomile has been used medicinally for thousands of years, dating back to the ancient Egyptians, Romans, and Greeks. But people with ragweed allergies should use it with caution.

Linda was a bit skeptical about herbs when she walked through my door, but all of her friends had come to me, and she didn't want to be left out. Her overall health was good, and she didn't suffer from excessive anxiety except when it came to her mother, who was in an assisted living facility. Paula had been an independent woman and had raised Linda to be one, too. But as Paula's health declined and her ability to care for herself became limited, Linda felt obliged to place her in a safe living arrangement. Paula would panic when it was time for Linda to go home. She wasn't on many medications, but refused to take an antianxiety pill, claiming it made her even more nervous.

I asked Linda whether she'd ever tried chamomile tea. She'd tasted it before but only as a light beverage—that is, the way most of us drink chamomile tea—a cup of water and one tea bag. I suggested that she up the ante in a daily late afternoon chamomile tea ritual with Paula using chamomile in medicinal strength—four teabags to a cup of water. I also suggested that she add a dropper of chamomile tincture to each cup, making the tea even stronger. This created a more concentrated and effective solution.

It worked out well! "I was making your tea daily for my mom but not really for myself," Linda told me. "I drank it with her so she wouldn't be drinking it alone. My mom really enjoyed it and said it made her feel better. She asked if she was allowed to have her chamomile tea twice a day! But what surprised me most was how it made me feel. Leaving my mother was always so painful, but after I drank the tea with her, I felt calmer—and so did she." At her follow-up, she shared other physical challenges she was having, saying, "If chamomile did magic for my nerves, I'm starting to believe in this 'herb-thing' my friends are raving about."

Chasteberry (*Vitex agnus-castus*) Used as a hormonal balancer for tension, agitation, lack of libido. It's specific to helping premenstrual anxiety and regulating the cycle.

Taylor knocked on my door. She had come to pick up herbs for a young child she was babysitting at the request of the child's mother. But I was so rude! I yanked this young woman into my office and said to her, "You're too beautiful to have such horrible acne." She was so offended by my directness. If eyes were daggers, she would have killed me on the spot! Clearly this was a sensitive issue for her, and she hated my guts for bringing it up.

But I persisted. I knew that I could help . . . so I asked Taylor what she'd done for her skin. "I've tried Retin-A," she told me, "and I've been to the dermatologist, but nothing worked." So, I asked her about her menstrual cycle. From her expression, I could tell that she was shocked that I—a stranger—had the audacity to pose such a personal question, but she answered me nonetheless. It turned out that her cycle was all over the place with little consistency. Most months, she didn't get her period. She would have cramps, breast tenderness, breakouts, but no menstrual bleeding. She had even tried birth control pills, but they made her sick. Her goal was to make peace with the terrible acne. That was that, but I was disturbing her resolve.

Again, I persisted. I looked at her skin with a magnifying glass and asked, "Have you ever tried herbal medicine? It may just be what you need right now."

I referred Taylor to my friend who does natural facials, and I put her on the herb chasteberry. Within twelve weeks, her skin looked remarkably better. The happy side effect was that her cycles were more consistent and, to her surprise, her moods were so much better. She had been unaware of how her skin problems and irregular cycle had affected her emotionally. She was all smiles when she came in for an herbal refill. "I am so much more in control of my mood swings," she told me. "It's really exciting, I can also pretty much predict my cycles, and I am confident with my skin challenges that are improving remarkably."

Chasteberry is a fabulous herb if your menstrual cycle is irregular. Extreme moodiness often comes on when a woman is anticipating her menstruation and it's delayed. During that "waiting time," you can feel edgy and agitated.

Damiana (*Turnera diffusa*) A nervine for women who are depressed, anxious, irritable, sad, and have extremely low libido.

Janet was referred to me after the birth of her second child because she was "stressed." She thought she was the only mother in the world who ever felt the pressure of having two young children at home. First, I confirmed that her emotions were normal and common. We discussed ideas for coping with the sleep deprivation and the physical stress she was experiencing. I suggested extra help around the house, possibly taking a gentle exercise class weekly, and going on an occasional date with her husband. That was when the tears started flooding.

"What is it?" I asked with concern. "Is your husband ill?"

"No," she sobbed. "It's me. I just don't feel sexual anymore. With the two kids, dishes, laundry, and dinners to cook and clean up after, I don't have the desire to be intimate."

I smiled and reassured her that she was certainly not alone with this feeling. "Many women during their childbearing years just can't find their 'sexy side.'" I told her. She asked me whether there was anything she could take, and I shared the good news that there is! "There's an herb called damiana that often helps women tap into their 'missing' desire. It's not a magic pill that will turn you into a vixen, but if taken three times a day over the next month (and with extra cleaning help), you and your husband may be pleasantly surprised."

Two months later at her follow-up appointment, Janet walked in, sat down, put on a gentle smile, and whispered, "Well I might not be the perfect sexual partner yet, but my husband wants to thank you for helping bring his wife back to him."

Damiana isn't an aphrodisiac; however, it's considered a sexual tonic that stimulates the intestinal tract and brings oxygen to the genital area. It also increases energy, which can do a lot to support libido and desire. For women, it often helps restore the ability to achieve orgasm. It begins to work over a series of weeks, not in a few hours like Viagra . . . so please be patient. Historically, damiana has also been used to relieve anxiety, nervousness, and mild depression. It's helpful for people who feel exhausted and burned out.

Eleuthero (*Eleutherococcus senticosus*) An adaptogen/nervine for women feeling burned out, agitated, angry, low libido, and exhaustion.

Leslie was an attorney—a type A personality—with an infant who was breastfeeding poorly. At two-and-a-half weeks postpartum, she was trying to maintain some of her high-end work functions from her home office. But her baby was crying, and she wasn't sleeping or eating properly. When she walked through my door, she was ready to have a nervous breakdown. Breastfeeding had worked without a hitch with her first child, so she assumed she could handle the second with no problem and go back to work. But babies are unpredictable and quite different from one another. And Leslie couldn't cope. She was feeling burned out—not a good state if you're nurturing a newborn.

I sat her down, gave her a warm cup of tea, pulled out my portable back-massage cushion, and told her we have to come up with a plan for her to not flame out. Part of it was to slow her down. I instructed her on the importance of eating real food, urged her to call her office to let them know she needed to take a six- to eight-week postpartum break, and taught her that this child needed to breastfeed in a different way than her first. I also brought the herb eleuthero into her life. And what a difference it made. In her next visit six weeks later, Leslie was the sophisticated, *calm* mom I had known her to be.

Eleuthero is for people who are burning the candle at both ends. It is part of a family of herbs called adaptogens that heal the whole body. (See Chapter 4.) Eleuthero is especially helpful for type A personalities who work too hard. This herb will help balance your adrenal glands and bring physical tone back into your nervous system. You will begin to feel its effects after a week, but it's advisable to use the herb for a minimum of three to six months and possibly for a year. It acts as a nervine (a category of herbs that specifically supports the nervous system and calms nerves) to improve the quality of sleep. It also helps people with chronic fatigue syndrome and adrenal fatigue. It increases endurance and stamina and speeds recovery. Athletes, but also women who have just given birth, benefit from it.

· · · · · · · · The Color of Herbs' Flowers? ·

Albert Einstein once said, "We still do not know one thousandth of one percent of what nature has." How true is that? For instance, we know colors, in general, have a big effect on our moods. In Chapter 11, I discuss that relationship when choosing clothes or house paint. But what about the colors of the herbs' flowers? Could they also affect our moods? For instance, do herbs with white flowers affect us differently than herbs with blue flowers? Kava kava, eleuthero, bacopa, and lemon balm all have white flowers and are used to calm the system, although in different ways. Are there similarities in the action of these plants due to their white flowers? We know that flowers' colors attract birds, bees, and other pollinators. Botanists and chemists study the chemical compounds in herbs, but no one, to my knowledge, has researched the colors of the flowers and whether they enhance the action of the herbs.

I called many distinguished herbalists to get their opinion. They all agreed this is an interesting hypothesis that warrants research. Matthew Wood, author of *The Earthwise Herbal Repertory*, told me, "The colors of flowers must have an influence on the way the herbs act in our bodies and minds but no research, to my knowledge, has been done in this area. There have been studies of the influence of colors. I find that red flowers are good for fever, blue is relaxing to spasms, lavender is relaxing to the nerves (rosemary, lavender, monarda), and burgundy builds the blood—it is the color of bone marrow and liver. Orange and yellow flowers are invigorating. The gentler, milder versions (pink, baby blue) may be the most soothing of all. They are associated with babies!"[6]

Herbalist Pam Montgomery, author of *Plant Spirit Healing*, told me, "We know that we see colors according to their vibrational energy and we also have different vibrational frequencies." We may not feel the vibration of the colors we see and we may not feel the vibrational energy as we ingest them, but that doesn't mean it doesn't affect us. Pam added another element: "I believe that plants and the plants, colors often correspond to the colors of the chakras."[7] So, when choosing an herbal protocol for a client, she looks at the colors in the plant and the chakra that needs assistance, and then finds an herb that matches.

Just for fun, here are the flower colors of some of the herbs I recommend:

Bacopa: white
Blue vervain: blue/purple
California poppy: orange
Chamomile: yellow
Chasteberry: purple/white
Damiana: yellow
Eleuthero: white
Fresh milky oats: white sap
Holy basil: pink
Lavender: purple
Lemon balm: white

Linden: yellow
Mimosa: pinkish
Motherwort: pink
Passion flower: purple, pink, blue
Rose: pink, red
Rosemary: purple
Saint-John's-wort: yellow; crushes to red
Skullcap: purple
Valerian: pink, white, red
Wild lettuce: yellow

Mood Herbs to the Rescue

Fresh milky oats (*Avena sativa, Avena fatua*) A nervine for women feeling burned out, grief-stricken, agitated, frazzled nerves, exhausted.

A client came in crying about everything . . . Melissa just wanted to do it all right. If her baby was happy, she'd be crying. If her baby was unhappy, she'd be crying. It was as if she were a walking open wound. Everything—negative or positive—stimulated the tears. She was afraid to sleep at night because she felt she had to watch her infant. Her nerves were shattered. She was hypersensitive and overprotective. But instead of helping her and her baby, this behavior was detrimental. She was falling apart.

Before races, horses are given oats because they calm the central nervous system but also rejuvenate energy. The same is true for us humans. So, we began by including fresh milky oats (these are oat seeds . . . not oatmeal) and twice-weekly walks in the park with her baby into Melissa's regimen. Fresh milky oats are great for women who experience anxiety and depression. They may suffer from insomnia, tension headaches, and emotional oversensitivity with outbursts of irritability and anger. Tears flow over the littlest things. Oats are a wonderful herb if you live with chronic stress; they can calm frazzled nerves. This herb is best when taken over a long period of time. You won't feel the effect right away, but be assured that it's doing its job. Think of fresh milky oats as a Band-Aid for your central nervous system. It's best used in combination with other herbs.

Melissa's blend used the oats as a base herb. She sometimes combined them with motherwort or skullcap. After a month, she returned for a follow-up appointment. "I've stopped crying about everything," she told me. "And my reactions are calming down." She was happy, and she loved that she could regulate herself with herbs. She was thrilled that she'd started losing the weight she'd gained during pregnancy—a lovely unintended consequence of her walking.

Holy basil (*Ocimum tenuiflorum*) An adaptogen/nervine for women with depression, anger, agitation, grief, sadness, and those who feel stuck.

Martha had given birth to ten children! She came to me with her last four kids for various breastfeeding issues and also for chronic yeast infections. A sophisticated woman and a teacher in her early fifties, she dreaded the upcoming parent-student conferences held twice a year at her school. She was embarrassed by her hot flashes. She was afraid her intermittent brain fog would prevent her from remembering all of her students' names.

She called me in desperation, saying, "I've seen five doctors already! I'm going crazy. I don't know what to do anymore."

Martha's medical odyssey began when her menstrual cycle started going haywire. She would bleed for ten days, be off for eight, and then bleed again for another fifteen. Sometimes the flow was heavy; sometimes it was light. She went to her general practitioner (GP) with these complaints, and he sent her to her gynecologist. "Oh, this isn't normal," he told her. He put her on birth control pills to regulate her cycle, but suddenly she developed severe headaches. The gynecologist sent her to a neurologist who gave her heavy-duty migraine medicine. During that meeting, she said, "I feel awful, and this whole thing is making me depressed." So, he sent her to a psychiatrist who put her on psychotropic and antianxiety medications. When she was in session with the psychiatrist, she complained about hot and cold flashes and dizziness. So, he sent her back to her general practitioner, who prescribed medication for inner ear problems to counteract her vertigo.

This would be comical if it weren't also true . . . and it was also terribly difficult for Martha. She started crying in my office. "I never took any medicine before," she told me as she laid out her five bottles of medications on my table. "What's going on with me?"

I pulled a well-worn book off my shelf, found a paragraph on perimenopause, and handed it to Martha to read. Within a few minutes, she was simultaneously sobbing and laughing. "I have every single symptom that a perimenopausal woman can have," she exclaimed. In the meantime, each of the doctors she'd seen told her she was sick. She wasn't sick at all. She was experiencing a normal hormonal transition, albeit a robust one. Once Martha understood she wasn't the only woman in the world going through this, we talked about many herbs she could take to ease her into menopause gracefully. She was so excited.

One I recommended was holy basil. Because of Martha's initial complaints of brain fog, I knew this might help her since it boosts cerebral circulation. This, in turn, improves memory and concentration. It's also an antistress herb that prevents excess adrenaline and cortisol production. A natural antidepressant, it enhances serotonin and dopamine levels. She took holy basil in combination with a few other herbs.

Knowing that her body's reaction was normal reduced Martha's anxiety significantly, and that accounted for 50 percent of the healing. My giving her other herbal choices put her in control. The herbs diminished her hot flashes and regulated the bleeding. I suggested other remedies for her migraines, and she made sure to take them at the onset of the headache . . . not when it was out of control. Since she started feeling better, and in consultation with her GP, she stopped taking the other medications. She was happy to have the herbs to "hold her hand" while she was going through the normal process of perimenopause, leading into menopause.

Kava kava (*Piper methysticum*) A nervine and sedative for women with muscle pain, trouble sleeping, agitation.

Joan was a hardworking medical resident who put 100 percent into everything she did. In addition to her continuing training, she was a wife and the mother of a small child. She was lucky that her supportive husband, mother, and mother-in-law were all on board to help raise her daughter and keep her house running smoothly. However, she put in long hours on her feet in the emergency room. When she finally came home after thirty-six-hour shifts, she would try her best to be a focused mom and loving wife, but it was tough. Crawling into bed, she knew she desperately needed sleep, but the tension in her body would not allow her to drift off. Instead, she tossed and turned. Her muscles were in knots from the hours she'd spent standing and leaning over patients. Her mind was also a whirl as she reviewed the patients she'd seen. She ended up reprimanding herself for the decisions she'd made that she now believed were wrong and reviewing the cases that were successful, tracing them step by step. This went on for hours. So, when the alarm went off, Joan was hardly refreshed. As the months passed, she became increasingly exhausted. After she told me her story, I could see that she was the perfect candidate for kava kava.

Kava kava (a.k.a. kava) has a long history as a gentle muscle relaxant. It relieves tension and clears stress from the mind. Used for hundreds of years in the Pacific Islands of Polynesia, it was a ceremonial drink that helped people ease the stresses of the day. The herb is not a psychedelic or hallucinogenic, as the press has purported, but is recommended by herbalists to calm the system. It's gentle, and when used in proper dosages, it can relieve the tight muscles, relax the mind, elevate the mood, increase feelings of well-being and contentment, and most important as regarded Joan, help the body and mind let go.

Joan was excited by what I told her. She loved the idea of incorporating this herb into her routine. I suggested that she take some, diluted in juice, during her dinner and then repeat the dose again a half hour before going to bed. After two weeks, Joan texted me, saying, "Thank you so much! With the help of kava kava, my body is learning how to relax when it needs to and my mind is not racing as much as it did. These days, I wake up feeling revitalized because I'm finally having the restful sleep I need."

Lavender (*Lavandula angustifolia*) An uplifting nervine for sadness, depression, feeling stuck, and grief.

Lavender is usually thought of as a lovely scent used as an essential oil, in bath salts, and in perfumes. But it has a remarkable history as an internal herb—in a tea, or my favorite way, as a tincture. It has been used for generations with much success in helping with sadness. Herbalist David Winston uses lavender for what he calls "stagnant" depression. This occurs when you feel mired in a negative state. You see very clearly what you want to achieve—the goals you want to accomplish—but you are emotionally paralyzed. Taking lavender as a tea or in tincture (rather than smelling it as an essential oil) can push you to open the door you feel has become nailed shut. It helps move you so you can get the help you need.

Jessica was a college student who couldn't find her major. She knew she was smart, but she became depressed and jealous of everyone around her. It seemed they all knew what they wanted to do, but she didn't. A general degree was not for her. She started pondering her future. "Maybe I shouldn't go to school. Maybe I should drop out." She started grieving her loss of direction and momentum and couldn't make a decision that would move her forward.

I recommended a combination of herbs for Jessica, but the heaviest was lavender. It removes cloudiness and doubt, and it helped this bright young woman break through her stagnant depression so she could consider more options and take the next step.

I am happy to report that Jessica decided to major in physical therapy with a specialty in sports injury. She had always been an avid athlete, but felt she wasn't good enough to be a professional. That's what sparked her depression and sadness. After using her herbal combination, Jessica realized that she could still be involved in sports by helping others heal from injuries and achieve their goals. At her follow-up appointments, she was eager to learn how she could eventually include herbs in her physical therapy practice, since she saw how much they helped her get out of her rut.

Lavender can simultaneously calm and uplift the body and mind. It supports the nervous system and digestive tract through its soothing properties. It also eases feelings of stress and agitation associated with women's cycles.

Mood Herbs to the Rescue

Lemon balm (*Melissa officinalis*) A calming nervine from the mint family, it was used as far back as the Middle Ages to reduce stress and anxiety, promote sleep, improve appetite, and ease pain and discomfort from indigestion.

Cindy was flying overseas with her three kids. She was always nervous planning a trip and getting to the airport. Her husband was a huge help, but when things got out of hand, he'd close down and fall asleep, which meant everything depended on her staying calm and being responsible. Cindy also discovered that her kids would get nervous because she was nervous. It would always turn into a vicious cycle!

She had seen herbs work wonders for her daughter if she had fluid in her ears. When she gave her son herbs for fever, he would feel calmer and heal more quickly. She wondered whether there were any relaxing herbs she could take and give to her kids before they traveled. I was happy to share lemon balm, an herb that's calming and soothing and safe for children. I suggested that she start taking the herb three times a day, the week before she was to travel. Her kids weren't having anticipatory anxiety, so she could start them the day before the trip when her tension would be rising and would rub off on them. The day of travel they all were to take it twice before the flight, three hours apart. I gave her some in a small bottle that she could bring on the plane, so she could take it as needed during the flight.

Lemon balm relieves stress without making you groggy. It also has antiviral properties, which are helpful when you're on a plane, breathing recycled air. It's in the mint family, so it's gentle with a slight lemon flavor. Although most of the herbs I use are in an alcohol base, lemon balm extracts well in glycerite, which doesn't need to be diluted for kids. It tastes amazing! Cindy was also excited to learn that this herb is wonderful for fevers, flu, and colds, and that it is the perfect addition to any mom's first-aid kit. Her trip was successful and she told me that she was already planning another one!

Linden (*Tilia americana, Tilia europea, Tilia cordata*) As a relaxing nervine, linden has been used for generations by people struggling with insomnia, nervous and muscle tension, anxiety, depression, and digestive issues originating from emotional unrest.

Monica always felt bloated after she ate. She came to me because she was a nurse in the emergency room and had to deal with and watch trauma every day. She was good at her job and knew how to act fast and be efficient, but by the end of her shift, her muscles ached and it was hard for her to digest food. She wasn't anxious, didn't suffer from panic attacks, and didn't feel particularly burned out. She just needed something she could turn to if the ER got too crazy and then later, after work, when she needed to wind down.

The way Monica described her life, I immediately knew she would fall in love with linden flowers. I had once learned from an herbalist who had a gorgeous garden in the back of her office, that she would take her clients out there, ask them to look at the herbs, and tell her which ones resonated with them. So, with Monica, I pulled out my phone and showed her a picture of a blooming linden tree. She looked at me, shocked. "Is that a medicinal tree? This is one of my favorites. It grows down the street from me. Every spring, I admire the flowers. Their smell is breathtaking and the petite flowers always grab my attention." She was excited to learn about this herb.

Monica liked linden flowers very much. She did have to change her diet and drink more water to alleviate her bloating, and I taught her a few exercises to relieve her sore muscles, but she carried this herb with her all the time and said that it took the edge off her stress at work. It helped calm her stomach after she saw tragedy. These small beautiful flowers are gentle and subtle but powerful.

Mimosa bark (*Albizia julibrissin*) A nervine used for sadness, depression, lack of libido, feeling stuck, and grief.

Mimosa bark is purported to bring joy to a person's heart. This herb is a mood elevator. Take it if you have a broken heart and can't get past it. I recommend it to many clients who feel stressed and overwhelmed toward the end of the day. Tammy knew, for instance, that her husband liked to go out to dinner and a movie every Thursday night. They enjoyed these dates. But if she had a conflict at work or her kids wouldn't settle down to their homework, she had trouble retrieving her loving feelings toward her husband. "I know I want to respond tenderly," she told me, "and I do adore Dave but . . ." Her moodiness got in the way.

Mimosa bark is traditionally associated with love. In the United States, when you love someone, you bring roses. In Europe and especially in Italy, it's customary to bring your loved one a bouquet of mimosa flowers. On the French Riviera, when the mimosa blooms transform the countryside with a golden haze each January and February, the Mimosa Festival celebrates these beautiful flowers. My clients know that if they want to feel the love at night, they will begin taking mimosa late in the afternoon. By the evening, it opens their heart and allows them to experience and express what they feel to their partner.

So, in a similar vein, why not treat yourself to the special present of mimosa bark if you are feeling sad, moody, or unloved? This herb can be used daily or occasionally as needed, but you don't have to limit it to only romantic encounters with your partner. Imagine your child is performing in a play at school. You're in a grumpy mood and know this will spoil your enjoyment and the connection to your budding actor. You can use mimosa bark to boost your loving feelings. It is a gentle but powerful herb.

Motherwort (*Leonurus cardiaca*) A nervine for women who feel gloomy (it's used for hormonal grumpiness or just grumpiness without the hormonal edge), a lack of libido, feeling stuck, agitation, and anger.

In Chapter 1, I explained how important motherwort has been to me personally and also professionally. In fact, this is my all-time favorite herb to help stabilize moodiness. Its effects can be felt within twenty minutes of taking it. Women of all ages and stages of life can benefit from it. Motherwort is wonderful for taking that "edge" off your more negative emotions and is helpful if you suddenly feel that "black cloud" descending. You can take it preventively if you know you will be encountering a difficult time or if you determine from your calendar that menstruation is approaching. After that, many women choose to use it as needed. My motto: *Motherwort—don't leave home without it.*

Passion flower (*Passiflora incarnata*) A nervine and sedative for women with insomnia, sadness, agitation, and grief.

Rebecca came in complaining of severe nausea and insomnia during her first pregnancy. She tossed and turned all night. I gave her a homeopathic remedy and also suggested the herb passion flower. I told her to take it with her dinner at six p.m. and then also at eight and eleven p.m.

Rebecca called before her follow-up appointment six weeks later. "I don't know if I should come back," she told me. "I don't know if anything is working. The nausea is 70 percent better, but I'm still nauseous." This is not unusual. Nausea with pregnancy is pretty hard to eradicate, and a 70 percent improvement is an amazing result with homeopathy. We can't get to 100 percent because nausea is usually an indication of a healthy pregnancy.

"I'd really like you to come back because I need to assess your case," I told her. When she came in, my first question was: "What's happening with your sleep problems?"

"What sleep problems?"

"You came to see me because you couldn't sleep," I reminded her.

"I did?" Rebecca was incredulous.

So, I showed her my notes. On every page, I'd written, "Can't sleep. Tossing and turning. Losing her mind." She was so anxious when she first saw me.

"Oh my gosh!" Rebecca said. "I didn't remember that!" The passion flower was working so well on her insomnia, she literally forgot it was one of the reasons she had come to see me.

Passion flower is a slight sedative. It's a nervine used for anxiety, insomnia, and nervous headaches. It's so gentle, it's safe enough to take during pregnancy. It helped Rebecca's mood and calmed her. Rather than tossing and turning in bed all night, she now awoke refreshed.

> **Rhodiola (*Rhodiola rosea*)** This adaptogen boosts the nervous system and has antidepressant qualities. It's not a stimulant per se, but it can enhance immunity, elevate the capacity for exercise, improve memory, and increase sexual function and energy.

Yolanda had been an athlete at college, on the tennis and soccer teams. She'd always prided herself on being fit and in shape. She was muscular but had to watch her weight. She came to me right after she'd finished law school saying, "I gained some pounds with all the hours sitting in the library, studying. I also snacked too much and didn't make time for meals. I didn't sleep enough, either. And now I'm burned out and foggy. I don't know how I passed the bar the first time I took it. This should be the happiest time in my life, but I feel as if I'm headed toward depression!" Yolanda looked as if she was about to burst out in tears, but she was too tired to cry. She also confided in me that she had just broken up with her long-term boyfriend because he wasn't willing to work on fixing their relationship.

Oh, boy! Adding all this up, the herb rhodiola was a no-brainer. It had been used in the Soviet Union for generations for athletes who got burned out and needed a boost. It has additional benefits as a brain tonic, increasing mental alertness and concentration in people who've studied too much and too long. Rhodiola has also been shown to be effective for cardiac problems caused or aggravated by stress. This was not an issue for Yolanda at her young age, but being that she has a type A personality, I warned her to take it easier. As an herbalist, my goal is to teach my clients how to prevent potential problems as well as solve their acute issues. I suggested she use the herb three times a day for a month and get back to me. I pointed out that since rhodiola has a slight stimulating property, she should not take it in the evening. We also talked about how she could resume her exercise routine.

Well, we all love success stories, and Yolanda is one of them. After one month, with taking the herb, getting more sleep, and going back to the gym, her spark reappeared. She opened a law practice with a colleague from school, and last I heard, she was engaged!

Rose (*Rosa damascena*) An uplifting nervine for women with sadness, stuck feelings, agitation, depression, grief, and gloominess.

Rose is used to alleviate emotional pain. I recommend it to women who are stuck in the feelings of a situation—they've been hurt, they experience injustice, they feel the world is unfair, they're in turmoil. Roses can help create a feeling of well-being.

My client Mary was residing in a city she didn't want to live in. She missed her family and friends—her old support system. Her husband's company had relocated him to this town. It was a great opportunity for advancement—so, there was little choice. Still, Mary acted as if she had raw skin. Everything bothered her. "How am I going to live here?" she lamented. "What did I do to deserve this?" Despite her unhappiness, she had to make peace with her situation because that's where she had to be.

I recommended rose to Mary because it can also bring joy to the heart. However, I coupled the remedy with the suggestion that she seek out a good psychotherapist. She needed more support to make her situation work.

Mary began taking the herb daily. She slowly felt her hardened heart melt, pumping new warmth into her system. She had never been a fan of roses but saw that the herb was moving her into the direction she wanted to go. She suddenly became attracted to roses and laughed as she told me, "I'm buying roses and putting them on my dining room table and in my kitchen. I even bought rose jelly for my morning toast. I figured if the herb helped me so much from the inside out, why not also have it around me from the outside in." She called me regularly to update me on the exciting new activities she was finding in the city she was forced to live in. She joined a gym and a book club and found charity organizations—all of which helped her acclimate to the town and make new friends. With the aid of botanicals, she had made the necessary adjustments and was no longer feeling victimized by her frustration.

> **Rosemary (*Rosmarinus officinalis*)** This herb can bring feelings of well-being and increase energy. It's known as an antidepressant and a soothing tonic for the nerves, which makes it excellent for people who deal with anxiety and depression. It also increases blood circulation to the brain, assisting with memory.

There are many reasons that I use rosemary in blends but rarely alone. The first is its strong taste. This herb helps with memory. Students studying for tests famously use the essential oil of rosemary to push circulation toward the brain. For anyone not so proficient at headstands, I recommend this herb because who couldn't benefit from a little more blood flow to the brain? Rosemary has been used for thousands of years and was known by ancient healers as an overall tonic for the nervous system. This herb can be added to any herb mentioned in this chapter if memory and brain fog have been a challenge.

> **Saint-John's-wort (*Hypericum perforatum*)** A nervine for women with muscle pain, sadness, depression, and agitation.

Saint-John's-wort is one of the most commonly used herbal products in the United States. In recent years, it has been studied extensively as a treatment for depression. According to the University of Maryland Medical Center, "Most studies show that St. John's wort may help treat mild-to-moderate depression, and has fewer side effects than most other prescription antidepressants. But it interacts with a number of medications, so it should be taken only under the guidance of a health care provider."[8] In particular, there is some concern about interactions of Saint-John's-wort with other psychotropic medications, so caution is advised.

Jenny came into my office wearing a bright yellow shirt and a big, toothy grin. She was extremely organized and punctual as well as polite and kind. But her smile was a dead giveaway. She was just too happy, too rehearsed. I could tell that behind the smile and bright appearance, she was gritting her teeth in pain.

I calmly began taking her history, waiting for her to reveal what was really going on. At first, she told me, "Oh, everything is fine," but soon her litany of symptoms began to snowball. "You know, I'm feeling a teeny tiny bit depressed," she said. "Just a tad gloomy and down. In general, I'm a happy person, but recently the littlest things get under my skin. And now, I'm getting random pains down my arms and in my jaw and have tension and muscle pain in my neck and shoulders."

All of Jenny's symptoms screamed out to me that she needed Saint-John's-wort, which is used both in a homeopathic and an herbal form. The homeopathic remedy is recommended for severe nerve pain that occurs with crushed fingers, toothaches, or pinched nerves. In fact, it's one of the most successful homeopathic agents for this kind of pain. In the herbal form, Saint-John's-wort works well for depression and especially for the type that makes a person feel as if she has raw skin that's constantly being rubbed. She may feel hypersensitive, sensorially agitated; sounds, lights, and even textures can be irritating. Saint-John's-wort also has a long history for the treatment of muscular pain, spasms, and cramps even with no depression.

The Saint-John's-wort plant has a beautiful bright-yellow flower that when crushed and made into an herbal remedy turns a deep red—much like the pain I felt had been lurking under Jenny's sunny appearance. I suggest that she take Saint-John's-wort internally and get weekly massages with the oil of the Saint-John's-wort flower. After a month of these treatments, Jenny began to feel much better and she fell madly in love with this herb.

Skullcap (*Scutellaria lateriflora*) A nervine for women with agitation, anger, sadness, insomnia, rage, and fear.

Laurie brought her youngest child to me so I could treat his chronic ear infections. She was one of the sweetest women I'd ever met. I loved the way she talked to her kids . . . she was so kind and responsible. So, imagine my shock when she blurted to me, "I am the worst mom in the world," during a follow-up visit.

"Can't be!" I said. "I was going to give you the award for the best mom of the month."

She shook her head. "As soon as my kids wake up in the morning, my heart starts racing and my stomach is churning. I'm so nervous and short-tempered. Every time a child has a request, I want to scream." Laurie felt super responsible that her three kids be clean, properly dressed, and well fed. She made sure they brushed their teeth and got to school on time. She fussed over her husband and always packed him a nutritious brown-bag lunch. She needed her bills to be paid and her house to be perfect when she left for work in the morning, too. All of this made her a serious nervous wreck.

Laurie had never had an outburst with her children or partner, but by keeping a lid on her emotions, she feared she would drop dead from the tension. She was sure her kids could feel what was going on inside her even though she kept smiling and acting kind. She feared she was damaging them from all the pressure she was feeling. She was unable to sleep at night, plagued by negative thoughts and guilt. "I don't know how long I can keep up the facade," she told me, wiping away tears.

We spent time discussing how Laurie's feelings are normal. "That's how lots of mothers of three young kids feel," I assured her, validating her emotions. And I told her that when it comes to her kids, "actions speak louder than thoughts." I also gave her a bottle of skullcap. She took the tincture three times a day. Within two weeks, she called me back. "This is the first time in years that I've actually enjoyed my children," she told me. "I don't feel the anxiety in my body anymore." Laurie sensed her central nervous system relaxing. She was calmed. She was a new person.

Once I told her how normal her feelings were, she began discussing her emotions with her friends. Soon she discovered that three quarters of the other moms felt exactly the way she did. And here she'd thought there was something really wrong with her!

I recommend skullcap for nervous tension with anxiety, nervous exhaustion, and stress headaches. It is considered a nervine and is used to counteract insomnia, anxiety, muscle tightness, and mild forms of obsessive-compulsive disorder. You will feel skullcap working within twenty minutes of ingestion. It's best used before an intimidating experience like a business meeting you've been anticipating for weeks, or right before it's time to put the children to bed. Skullcap can be taken over a long period or as needed. There has been some question about whether this herb should be combined with psychotropic drugs, so consult with an herbalist if you are currently taking these medications.

Valerian (*Valeriana officinalis*) A nervine for women with depression, anger or rage, agitation, muscle pain, or insomnia.

I recommend valerian to women who tend to get angry, feel resentful, or believe they have a heavy emotional burden that makes it difficult for them to move around. One of my clients, Dina, loved her kids but everything they did made her mad. In fact, she was angry, exhausted, and stressed out all the time. She was able to control herself around her kids, but boy, was she yelling inside. She didn't spare her husband. She would lash out at him when he came home late. Her tension was so high, she experienced muscle spasms and headaches. And she was not enjoying restful sleep. Her goal was to get into bed by ten. But often, she wouldn't make it until eleven p.m. or later because there was too much to do. And then, she'd lie there angry and upset for the next two hours, ruminating on how she'd be incapacitated the following day. It became a vicious cycle—one that Dina didn't know how to break.

The first thing we talked about when she came in was hiring a cleaning lady to help her with the burden of the household. I spoke to her about some simple, healthful dinner ideas that would free up more time. We talked about adding regular exercise to her routine. And I suggested valerian.

Valerian improves sleep quality with no daytime sedation or impairment of concentration or performance. It can reduce night awakening, and in a randomized study, it was as effective as Oxazepam (an antianxiety medication) for sleeping.[9] It eases muscle pain and decreases tension headache, anxiety and irritability, nervous stomach, and other stress-induced gastrointestinal symptoms.

Although Dina had been skeptical at first about herbs helping her out of her rut, six weeks later, she had to admit that not only had her sleep improved, but her daily rages had decreased significantly. She could honestly say she was beginning to enjoy her kids. And fortunately for everyone, she had stopped berating her husband.

Wild lettuce (*Lactuca virosa*) A sedative used as a sleep aid and a pain reliever.

I recommend wild lettuce to women who not only have trouble falling asleep, but can't stay asleep. It also relieves muscle pain, muscle spasms, arthritis, stomachache, and emotional pain. Although it is not used specifically as an herb to help with moodiness, I often add wild lettuce to blends. This herb is in the opiate family, but isn't addictive and doesn't have side effects, unless you think reducing muscle pain and getting a good night's sleep is a side effect.

THERE ARE SO many herbs to choose from! I'm sure with some patience and time, you'll land on the one (or ones) that are perfect for your situation.

Finally, in your quest for Moodtopia, you can employ one more element—that of your sense of smell. In the next chapter, we'll explore the many mood-related benefits of essential oils and aromatherapy.

CHAPTER SIX

AROMATHERAPY: SCENTS-ING YOUR WAY TO SERENITY

Smell is a potent wizard that transports you across
thousands of miles and all the years you have lived.

—HELEN KELLER

Can different scents help you feel better emotionally and control your moods? You bet—just think about the lift you get when you wear your favorite perfume or inhale the comforting aroma of a tray of hot chocolate-chip cookies coming out of the oven—a favorite when you were a kid.

Aromatherapy is the use of essential oils that, in therapeutic doses, promote physical, emotional, and spiritual health. The good news is that essential oils come in tiny vials that fit in the palm of your hand so they're easy to carry in your purse, wallet, or the basket of your stroller. You can even slip one in your bra or sock.

The French chemist and perfumer René-Maurice Gattefossé first coined the term *aromatherapy* in 1937. He wasn't a believer or practitioner of the natural health movement, but as a chemist, he was interested in essential oils' properties. In 1910, he burned his hand badly in his laboratory. It being the first compound handy, he grabbed undiluted lavender oil to pour over his skin. He was shocked to find that it not only instantly eased the pain, but helped heal his hand without infection or scars. He went on to discover that minute amounts of essential oils are absorbed by the body and interact with its chemistry.[1]

Since the late 1970s and early '80s the use of essential oils and aromatherapy has become a major part of alternative and holistic health systems. It has a huge following across the world and in the United States. But other cultures throughout history have used these oils for therapeutic purposes for over five thousand years. The ancient Chinese, Indians, Egyptians, Greeks, Romans, and Jewish cultures employed them in cosmetics, perfumes, hygiene, therapy, for spiritual and ritualistic purposes, and even as medicines.

In this chapter, I'll teach you how to create your own mood-enhancing therapeutic scent tool for your home, car, office, hotel—wherever. You can even use it preventively. If you know you're going on a long car ride that will make you grumpy, then diffusing certain essential oils in the car will help you feel happier. If you are nervous boarding a plane, dab some essential oil on a tissue and inhale it as needed throughout the trip. If you are typically grouchy early in the morning, but you'd rather start your day off on the sunny side of the street, use some stimulating scents.[2]

Prevention is always best, but in a moment of crisis, essential oils can be an important tool to help you achieve Moodtopia. They support and enhance your body's innate healing response. Using aromatherapy to relieve moodiness, anxiety, and stress and to dispel worry and panic is enjoyable and easy.

HOW DO ESSENTIAL OILS AND AROMATHERAPY WORK?

Essential oils help your moods because they have properties that, when inhaled or applied topically, work on the sympathetic and parasympathetic nervous systems and promote serotonin and dopamine secretion.

When you sniff something, the olfactory (smell) receptors in your nose send a signal to the olfactory bulb in your brain. This is where you perceive smell. The olfactory bulb then signals other areas of the brain including the limbic system. The latter has been called the primitive part of the brain. It controls instinct, mood, and such emotions as anger, anxiety, depression, and joy. It also controls drives, such as hunger, sex, dominance, protection, and care for children. The limbic system can directly activate the hypothalamus, which acts as a hormone control center (ever heard of hormonal moodiness?). It governs growth, sex, and thyroid hormones as well as neurotransmitters such as serotonin, which helps to mediate depression.

Our sense of smell is our only sense that's wired directly to the limbic system. But what's interesting is that when it comes to smell, we react instantaneously and think later. Have you ever had the experience of a scent's triggering memories and emotions so vividly that it feels as if you are there? Maybe the aroma of coffee in the morning reminds you of the security you felt seeing your father sitting at the kitchen table as you ran off to school. Or a pumpkin pie in the oven evokes Thanksgiving dinners during which you loved playing with your cousins; you get a jolt of pleasure whenever you smell cinnamon and cloves.

Since odors have a direct path to the limbic system, what you smell (including essential oils used in aromatherapy) has a profound effect on your moods and emotions. Rachel S. Herz, an assistant professor of psychology at Brown University, teaches that "no other sensory system has this type of intimate link with the neural areas of emotion and associative learning, therefore there is a strong neurological basis for why odors trigger emotional connections."

Studies with children have shown that fetuses learn odors even before birth! "Flavor compounds from the maternal diet get incorporated into amniotic fluid and are ingested by the developing fetus," Dr. Herz explains. "In studies where mother's consumption of distinctive smelling substances such as garlic, alcohol or cigarette smoke were monitored during pregnancy, it was found that their infants preferred these smells compared to infants who had not been exposed to these scents."[3]

OUR CONDITIONED RESPONSES

Clearly, we associate certain odors with events in our life that were safe, healing, and pleasurable. The same can be true of painful experiences. This is quite individual. For instance, the smell of burning wood can evoke warm scenes beside the hearth or a burned-down home.

In the long run, odors affect our moods, work performance, and behavior because of their association with an event in our life. Herz writes, "We know that the neurological substrates of olfaction are especially geared for associative learning and emotional processing." One event becomes linked to another because of your past experiences. "The linked event is then able to elicit a conditioned response for the original situation," she explains.[4]

Essential oils are useful for "associative learning." For instance, imagine your child, Sophia, has trouble falling asleep. If you expose her to lavender oil every night when you're readying her for bed, she will connect the scent with sleep. Even if Sophia resists lying down, her brain will make conscious and unconscious associations with sleep. Her body will assist, and she'll doze off. Likewise, say that you are always stressed around your brother-in-law John. You can't remove him from your life, but you can practice deep-breathing exercises while inhaling a soothing essential oil. This can teach your body to calm itself. If you do this exercise consistently before you see John, eventually simply smelling the scent will automatically quiet your responses.

Because of the context, essential oil aromas are individual to each person. A particular scent that helps one woman with moodiness may cause agitation in another. In this chapter you'll read some guidelines, but if you don't like an oil that's purported to help with stress, then it's not for you. Oils used in healing are different than those in perfumes. The former must be of a therapeutic strength, pure, and naturally extracted. In the perfume business, synthetic products may be added to the oils, contaminating them to some degree.

DO ESSENTIAL OILS REALLY HELP US?

Few reliable scientific studies have been conducted, but one at the Mie University School of Medicine in Japan found that patients with depression needed smaller doses of antidepressant medications after citrus fragrance treatment.[5] Another study at the University of Vienna demonstrated that when the scent of orange oil was used in dental clinics, female patients exhibited decreased anxiety.[6] These investigations suggest that some fragrances may have a clinically quantifiable effect on mood.

Another explanation for mood improvements and reported pain reduction may be the placebo effect. According to this theory, an individual's expectations, rather than the scent's characteristics, determine the effects of the scent. Several studies conducted at the Monell Chemical Senses Center in Philadelphia found that subjects who were informed that an odor would improve performance achieved better results in a series of math calculations. These studies show that people's expectations about fragrances have the power to affect their health and behavior.[7] I've seen in my practice that the oils really do have an effect on people—but the emotional association has an impact, too. Perhaps the chemistry and the placebo effect work synergistically to help my clients.

HOW ARE ESSENTIAL OILS MADE?

Essential oils are derived from fragrant or aromatic plants, especially flowers, but also from buds, sap, leaves, twigs, seeds, roots, wood, and grasses. Most pure essential oils have been extracted through steam distillation. The essential oil is collected and bottled in small amber or blue vials to keep out sunlight, which would cause it to deteriorate. A by-product of this distillation is the remaining water. Some plants contain aromatic compounds that are so water soluble, they remain in these waters. These are quite fragrant and are called hydrosols. Aromatherapists use them, especially to moisturize skin.

Many companies employ chemical solvents to distill the essential oils, but most aromatherapists don't like this process. They're concerned that slight traces of the solvent may remain, even though they're supposed to be removed. That is why it's important to look for the term *pure* when you purchase your oils.

There are a few major companies around the world that make essential oils and most producers buy from them. Those I like: New Directions Aromatics, Aura Cacia, Snow Lotus, Doterra, Young Living, Mountain Rose Herbs, Art Naturals, and Plant Therapy.

CHOOSING AN ESSENTIAL OIL

These products come in the form of a single oil or a blend (of usually three to eight oils). Visit a health food store and experiment with smelling different single extractions and some blends. Or order an essential oil sampler packet online. The best samplers are from Snow Lotus, which has good, safe oils that I trust. Note: You may want to grab a bag of coffee beans in the store or have beans on hand to breathe between fragrances or if you have a hard time identifying which fragrances you prefer. Studies show coffee helps clear the nose and allows you to properly experience the next scent.[8]

Have some fun with smells and find a few oils you like, then begin to experiment with them and discover which essential oils help you with your moodiness. Single oils are wonderful, and premade blends can be divine. Once you become familiar with essential oils and use them, you can begin to make your own blends and create ones specific to your own personal needs.

A Note on the Notes . . .

Essential oils are classified by their "notes," which refer to their scent characteristics. Top notes tend to evaporate more quickly and are light and fresh, whereas middle notes are warm and soft fragrances that give body to a blend and have a balancing effect. Base notes, on the other hand, are heavier, solid, and intense. They are richly scented and relaxing in nature.

Persephenie, a perfumer based in Los Angeles, explains that when you smell essential oils, "you can sense a top, middle, and base note in your body. With direct inhalation, top notes are bright and uplifting, and you can feel their effect in your head. Top notes tend to vitalize and help battle mental fatigue. Middle notes, or 'heart' notes, are felt in your chest. Flowers are typically middle notes known to open and heal the heart. They are wonderful for addressing such issues as sadness and loss. Base notes are deep and are felt in the lower abdomen. Roots and woods fall in this category, and inhalation of a base note may help one feel grounded, stable, and rooted to the earth."[9]

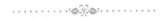

The following are commonly used to help with moodiness.

- **Basil** (*Top note: sweet, herbaceous, licorice-like, slightly camphorous*) Basil oil is energizing. It can stimulate your mind and help you focus on the tasks you're struggling with. Basil can easily dominate a blend, so use it sparingly.
- **Bergamot** (*Top note: flowery, fruity*) Bergamot oil has an uplifting effect that can alleviate anxiety, depression, and sadness or grief. It is purported to help work out fears of rejection or not being good enough. It can help you find your authenticity so you don't spend so much time worrying about what others think. It also helps in processing and releasing fear, criticism, shame, emotional pain, feelings of inadequacy, inferiority, or worthlessness. It helps you step into your own confidence and find joy.
- **Birch** (*Middle note: woodsy, herbaceous*) Birch oil is remarkable for muscle pain and is also used for inflammation and circulation. Since it has all these qualities for the body, it

also helps with pain in your mind. The oil is stimulating and promotes feelings of strength, warmth, and vitality. It can assist you in finding your own inner support and strength, rooting yourself into your own center.

- **Black pepper** (*Middle note: spicy*) This is stimulating and usually used in combination with other oils to enhance alertness and increase stamina. Avoid it before bedtime.

- **Chamomile, German** (*Middle note: herbaceous, sweet, fruity*) This calms the nerves and supports digestive health. The German variety excels in the treatment of irritated skin. Chamomile is also often used to treat depression.

- **Chamomile, Roman** (*Middle note: herbaceous, sweet, fruity*) Calms the nerves and supports digestive health. The Roman variety is superior in addressing mental anxiety, paranoia, and hostility. Chamomile is also often used to treat depression.

- **Cedarwood** (*Base note: fresh, woody, balsamic*) Cedarwood oil is said to have a grounding, calming effect on the nervous system and is thought to bring people together spiritually. It may help individuals feel strong and confident in themselves, while at the same time enabling them to reach out for connection and support from those around them. This oil both roots a person and opens his or her heart.

- **Cinnamon** (*Middle note: spicy, earthy*) You can buy either cinnamon bark oil or cinnamon leaf oil. They have similar properties, though the bark oil is stronger. Cinnamon is warming, stimulating, and energizing and is used to reduce drowsiness and irritability. Diffused at home on a cold winter's day, it brings joy. It blends well with many other essential oils, especially oils in the wood, spice, citrus, and mint families.

- **Clary sage** (*Top note: earthy, herbaceous, subtly fruity*) Clary sage oil is used to relieve muscle and nervous tension. It also has the ability to help with "clarity," giving you the ability to see what was muddled and to help you look ahead with vision. It is often used during meditation, contemplation, and creative work. It can help you when you get lost in your own thoughts and need to tap into something deeper. It helps open you to intuition and inner wisdom.

- **Clove** (*Middle note: spicy, warming yet slightly bitter, woody*) Clove oil is strong and must be used with caution. It is nature's painkiller. It's said to promote healthy boundaries, helping one feel empowered to stand strong and break patterns of victimization by enhancing the ability to speak up for oneself. Some practitioners use it for people who are struggling with codependency.

- **Cypress** (Middle note: fresh, herbaceous, slightly woody) Cypress oil is a stimulant used to treat low blood pressure and poor circulation. Use it if you feel exhausted all the time and find it difficult to concentrate.

- **Eucalyptus** (Top note: fresh, woody, earthy) This is a medicinal oil used to treat flu, fever, and sore throat. Emotionally, it relates to a person's willingness to be well. Many people have underlying patterns that keep them perpetuating illness. Eucalyptus oil can help them regain their own health and empower them to allow themselves to get healthy. It can even help change past patterns that may keep a person in the role of victim.

- **Fir needle** (Middle note: fresh, woody, earthy, sweet) Fir needle oil smells like Christmas trees and often evokes happy memories. It can also help people feel grounded and support those who feel inadequate. It is relaxing and calming and makes one feel safe.

- **Frankincense** (Base note: fresh, woody, balsamic, slightly spicy and fruity) This oil is used in meditation and ceremonies. It promotes deep breathing and relaxation, which can open nasal passages and reduce blood pressure, calming the system. With its comforting, warm, exotic aroma, it works as a sedative that induces feelings of peace, relaxation, satisfaction, and spirituality.

- **Geranium** (Middle note: floral, fresh, sweet) Geranium oil helps people who have been deeply hurt and struggle with sadness and overwhelming emotions. It can help them express their emotions and regain their trust in the world. For others, it tears down barriers and helps release anger.

- **Ginger** (Base note: warm, spicy, earthy, woody) Ginger oil is warming, energizing, and uplifting and is considered by some an aphrodisiac. It has also been called the "oil of empowerment," countering feelings of powerlessness and reducing fear in the body. It can create an inner fire and helps you walk into the role of leader in your own life so you stop feeling victimized.

- **Grapefruit** (Top note: citrusy, clean, fresh) This is a wonderfully energizing oil that's not too overpowering. I love diffusing it in the morning or when I need a bit of a boost. It has a wonderfully cleansing scent that has an uplifting effect on the mood and can bring joy to the heart. This oil can also assist with stress and depression.

- **Jasmine** (Middle note: warm, floral, exotic) Jasmine oil is also uplifting and has been used to help combat depression because of these properties. It can produce feelings of confidence and optimism. It will revitalize your energy and help you center yourself so you can find your inner support and strength. Jasmine is considered an aphrodisiac and is one of the most potent oils to boost depleted sexuality. It may also help when you're feeling scattered, overwhelmed, and generally stressed.

- **Juniper berry** (*Middle note: crisp, woody, sweet, earthy*) This oil is calming and eases stress without being a sedative. It's considered a spiritual oil and is a good choice during prayer or meditation. It gives you the strength to dig deep and face your fears so you can heal them. (Facing your fears is the only way to get rid of them.) It is also helpful with nightmares in adults and children and promotes more restful sleep.

- **Lavender** (*Top/middle note: floral, fresh, sweet, herbaceous*) This is said to be the oil of honest communication and expression. It's well known for its sedative properties and is used worldwide to induce peaceful sleep. It also calms a racing mind. Lavender has a balancing effect, and if used during the day, can be gently uplifting. Emotionally, it also eases anxiety and allows a person to feel present, calm, and engaged with a sense of peaceful security.

- **Lemon** (*Top note: fruity*) This is an uplifting and perky oil. These effects awaken the senses, clear the mind of distractions, and help a person tune in to the task at hand—so it promotes concentration. It can reduce anger and anxiety, promote focus, and dispel exhaustion. Lemon can clear the air when tension and anger has filled the space. Emotionally and spiritually, it provides clarity. It helps a person overcome confusion or doubt, fatigue, overwhelm, and lack of enthusiasm. It clears self-doubt, limiting beliefs, stagnant energy, and rigidness in the mind, heart, or body.

Making Lemonade

Lemon (the fruit), lemon balm, lemongrass, and lemon verbena are four totally different plants that yield distinct essential oils.

Lemon essential oil is made by compressing the peel of the fruit.

Lemon balm, also called *Melissa officinalis,* is a member of the mint family.

Lemongrass essential oil is used as aromatherapy to relieve muscle pain, kill bacteria on the skin, ward off insects, and reduce body aches. Taken internally, it helps the digestive system.

Lemon verbena helps with stress and anxiety. It's extracted from the *Aloysia citrodora* plant.

- **Lemon balm** (*Top/middle note: fresh, lemony, herbaceous*) This calming oil is also uplifting to the mind and especially the spirit. It relaxes the body, mind, and soul while bringing peace and contentment. It has a history of use for anxiety, nervousness, shock, depression, hypertension, and insomnia. It helps promote restful sleep. This oil can teach us how to allow calmness to flow through us and our life again. It lifts us out of those dark places and back into light and hope.
- **Lemongrass** (*Top note: fresh, lemony, earthy*) Besides its being a delicious citrusy seasoning in Thai cooking, most of us would never guess that lemongrass holds so much healing power inside its fibrous stalks. This essential oil is used as a pain reliever. It's said to be the oil of energetic cleansing for your home and person. It helps you let go of negative energy if you feel stuck, heavy, or low.
- **Lemon verbena** (*Middle note: bright, citrusy, floral undertones*) Often found in skin-care products, this oil has soothing properties but can also be a subtle erotic stimulant. Uplifting, it can support mental and creative activity.
- **Lime** (*Top note: fresh, citrusy, sweet, slightly tart*) This is among the most affordable of essential oils and is routinely used for its energizing, fresh, and cheerful aroma. It's well known for its ability to cleanse, purify, and renew the spirit and helps ground the body by pulling the energies inward and centering an individual. It is also used to focus attention and relieve irritation, worry, and stress.
- **Patchouli** (*Base note: rich, earthy, woody*) Patchouli essential oil is said to have strong aphrodisiac properties and stimulates desire. It has been used to help impotence and loss of libido. This oil also helps you connect to your own body and not disassociate when feeling unbalanced. It relieves anxiousness and stress and helps dispel shame and incompleteness.
- **Peppermint** (*Top note: minty, fruity*) This is one of the most widely used aromatic oils. The oil of peppermint is uplifting, refreshing, and rejuvenating to both the heart

and mind. For many, it initiates good memories from childhood. It can help you rise above stress, pain, sadness, or fear, and ignite the fire to regain the sense of zest and joy for life. It is also used for someone experiencing grief, hopelessness, and even pessimism. It gives people the strength needed to manage what comes their way in a refreshing manner.

⊰ **Marjoram** (*Base note: herbaceous, woody, sweet, slightly camphorous*) This oil has been used to mask foul odors for generations. It symbolizes happiness and was called "joy of the mountains." The herb was given to new brides and grooms to insure good luck, calmness, and happiness. The oil also helps combat insomnia, anxiety, and stress.

⊰ **Myrrh** (*Base note: warm, earthy, woody, balsamic*) This oil has been used as incense in religious ceremonies since antiquity. It's considered a spiritual oil that brings inner peace, tranquility, foresight, and deep thinking.

⊰ **Neroli** (*Middle note: intensely floral, citrusy, sweet, exotic*) This is both a sedative and overall tonic to the nervous system. It can be beneficial for most stress-related challenges. It has been said to treat heart palpitations, relieve insomnia and depression, and reduce nervousness.

⊰ **Rose** (*Middle note: strongly floral, sweet*) This is a highly versatile essential oil, but the pure form is quite expensive, requiring sixty thousand roses for every ounce of oil. (You can buy less expensive versions.) This oil provides relief from stress, insomnia, and depression. Emotionally, rose oil eases the heart during times of grief. It can also help people who have a hardened heart and heal relationships. It's considered an aphrodisiac.

⊰ **Rosemary** (*Middle note: fresh, herbaceous, sweet*) Rosemary oil is refreshing and a stimulating pick-me-up. It's famous for improving memory retention, focus, and alertness. Because of rosemary's stimulating properties, it can fight physical exhaustion and mental fatigue. It's a good choice for blends if you're driving long distances or engaged in long study sessions. It promotes mental expansion, clarity, and insight, and therefore can be especially useful during transition and change. It helps us process what's happening around us and within us consciously, instead of burying issues with distractions. In so doing, it creates a sense of trust in the process of life and confidence in our ability to navigate it with ease.

⊰ **Sandalwood** (*Base note: rich, sweet, fragrant yet delicate, woody, floral*) This is widely known as a spiritual, sacred oil, used around the world during prayer and meditation. It calms a busy mind and helps you let go of worry, allowing you to relax into a peaceful state. It's used to relieve tension, stress, and low self-esteem. It's also considered an aphrodisiac.

⊱ **Spearmint** (*Top note: minty, slightly fruity*) Spearmint is a gentler fragrance, so it's used when peppermint is too strong. The oil is energizing, revitalizing, and encouraging. Many feel it inspires a sharpness of mind and confidence in sharing insights. It can lift one's mood, especially if suffering depression, stress, or mental exhaustion.

⊱ **Tangerine** (*Top note: fresh, sweet, citrusy*) This oil is uplifting and is known to enhance creativity. It encourages playfulness and happiness, allowing you to be lighthearted and live spontaneously. It can brighten up your mood if you feel overwhelmed and overworked.

⊱ **Tea tree** (*Middle note: fresh, woody, earthy, herbaceous*) This oil is called a "medicine cabinet in a bottle" because it can treat bacteria, fungi, and viruses and it stimulates the immune system. It's said to promote healthy boundaries in unhealthy or toxic relationships. It can also create balance and is especially helpful with codependency.

⊱ **Thyme** (*Middle note: herbaceous, earthy*) Associated with the kitchen, this energizing and revitalizing oil also has many aromatherapy applications. It has been used to promote courage and helps with focus and mental clarity. It has been used for generations to cleanse the environment and "cleanse" or move blocked or stuck emotions. It can also fight infections. Thyme was burned in Greek temples to sanctify and purify the environment.

⊱ **Vanilla** (*Base note: fruity*) Vanilla essential oil is said to be the closest in fragrance and flavor to mothers' milk. This oil has the ability to both soothe and relax the mind. It has a calming effect on the brain and the nerves that provides relief from anxiety, anger, and restlessness, but it also stimulates mental clarity.

⊱ **Vetiver** (*Base note: woody, smoky, earthy, herbaceous, spicy*) Vetiver essential oil is remarkably soothing and calming. This oil is quite strong on its own and it should be well diluted or blended with other oils. It can help ground you and is a good choice if you need to unwind or de-stress. It helps with anxiety, anger issues, exhaustion, and coping with fear or insecurity. Vetiver can promote restful sleep.

⊱ **Wild orange** (*Top note: citrusy, sweet*) Wild orange essential oil is very uplifting, cheerful and energetic to the mind and emotions, which can translate to an increase in physical energy. It can help elevate your mood, and can open your mind and heart to the potential that surrounds you. It may stimulate creativity, vision, and widen your perspective. The orange aroma is so playful and fun, it can also help you tap into your own playfulness and sense of humor, so that challenges can be approached without the heaviness that might impact your ability to navigate them.

- **Ylang-ylang** (*Middle/base note: flowery*) Ylang-ylang essential oil is used to relax both the mind and body. It has a simultaneous sedative and euphoric effect on the nervous system. It can also help slow rapid breathing and heartbeat. It has a unique fragrance and is used as an aphrodisiac. It will uplift moods and promote feelings of happiness and joy while reducing anxiety, nervousness, panic, and fear. In this way, it helps people cope with depression.

· · · · · · · · Which Oils to Choose ·

Many essential oils have a calming effect for moods and relieve stress and anxiety, whereas others are uplifting. Here are a few suggestions for specific issues:

+ **If you have insomnia, are waking frequently at night or feeling restless and tense during the day:** chamomile, marjoram, neroli, sandalwood, vetiver, or ylang-ylang.
+ **If you're feeling anxious and are unable to relax:** basil, bergamot, frankincense, geranium, jasmine, juniper, lavender, lemon balm, neroli, or ylang-ylang.
+ **If your anxiety has morphed into depression and you need an emotional pick-me-up:** bergamot, clary sage, geranium, grapefruit, lavender, lemon, or vetiver.
+ **If you're suffering from nervous tension, add a few drops of any of the following oils to a carrier oil and massage into the back of your hands:** bergamot, cedarwood, cinnamon, clary sage, geranium, jasmine, lavender, sandalwood, or ylang-ylang.
+ **If you're struggling with brain fog:** basil, eucalyptus, mint, peppermint, or rosemary.
+ **If you'd like to feel more sexual:** jasmine, neroli, patchouli, rose, or ylang-ylang.

· · · · · · · · · · · · · ·✦✿✦· · · · · · · · · · · ·

HOW TO USE YOUR OILS

When we think of aromatherapy, we think of breathing in oils. When we inhale a fragrance, the scent molecules waft up the nose where they are received by olfactory receptors. When you breathe in an essential oil through the nose, the tiny oil molecules in the vapor contain the same properties that the oil contains. Oil molecules inhaled through nose or mouth also move into the lungs and interact with the lungs and respiratory system and mind.

· · · · · · · · As a Precaution . . . ·

> Be sure to keep your eyes closed and do not get any essential oil into your eyes. If you do happen to do so accidentally, dilute immediately with a carrier oil, such as sweet almond or olive oil—never use water! It will burn quite intensely at first but will pass in a few minutes.
>
> **Important note: there are some essential oils you should avoid in baths.** Don't use spicy or strong oils in the bath as they can burn the skin. These include cinnamon oil, oregano oil, and thyme oil; phototoxic oils such as citrus, especially bergamot oil; and those with specific irritant potential, such as lemongrass oil.

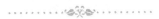

There are many ways to incorporate essential oils into your life to help with your moods. Why not try some of the following:

- **Bottle inhalation method:** Begin by holding the essential oil bottle at the level of your heart. Waft it and breathe deeply. If you like the scent and it seems appropriate, move it closer to your nose and breathe more deeply. If not, move onto another oil.
- **Hand inhalation method:** This is a wonderful method if you need a quick and easy way to stabilize your moods. Place 1 or 2 drops of oil on your palms, rub them together gently to activate it, then cup your hands over your mouth and nose. Breathe gently at first, and then, if you bond with the scent, breathe deeply,

imagining the scent going into your lungs. However, do this only with oils that can be safely applied directly to the skin (what we call "neat") without a carrier oil. (I explain this more extensively in the sidebar "I'll Have Mine 'Neat,'" page 103.)

- **Drop on pillowcase:** This helps you fall asleep or just de-stress at night. Put a few drops on the outer edges of your pillow, parallel to each other. Whether you roll to the right or left, you will inhale the fragrance. Use an inexpensive pillowcase that you don't mind staining, as carrier oils will discolor fabric. This method also works well with children.

- **Use a cotton ball or handkerchief:** Many of my clients who experience anxiety in school or work would never pull out a bottle and start sniffing it. In this case I suggest putting drops of essential oil on a tissue and leaving it in your pocket or purse. When you feel stressed, pull it out and take a few deep inhalations. Or you could keep a cotton ball infused with drops of essential oil in a resealable plastic bag. It traps the fumes. All you need to do is open the bag and take a whiff. Business-people can carry a handkerchief in their pocket and wipe their nose, inhaling the oils throughout the day.

- **Steam bowl inhalation:** This is a direct and intense method. The steam quickly vaporizes the oil. It's rapidly absorbed into the throat, sinuses, and then bloodstream. You'll need a stainless-steel or tempered glass bowl. Fill the vessel with filtered, boiled water (you don't want any chlorine) and add no more than 1 to 2 drops of your chosen essential oil to it—more than that can be overwhelming. Close your eyes or use swimming goggles as a protection (yes, your kids or roommates may laugh at you). Place a towel over your head, lean over the bowl, and breathe deeply. Don't burn yourself!

- **Facial steam machines:** Cute machines to steam your face for a home-facial are available online. They often have a plastic part to place your face in. These also work beautifully for aromatherapy. The same rules apply as with steam bowl inhalation.

- **Candle diffuser:** You will need to add water to the top of the dish or receptacle to fill or nearly fill it. Add 6 to 8 drops of essential oil to start. The candle is placed beneath the water—otherwise heat from a candle would be too intense and would burn the oil and not vaporize it. You may find you need more or less oil, depending on the type and strength of the oil and the size of the room. But please be careful. These oils are flammable.

- **Cool air nebulizing diffuser:** This system uses air pressure generated by a compressing unit to vaporize the essential oils. A glass nebulizing bulb serves as a condenser, allowing only the finest particles of the essential oil to escape. Gorgeous diffusers are sold online.

- **Terra-cotta pendant method:** Put a drop of oil on a terra-cotta pendant, fasten it around your neck (oil side facing out), or hang it from the rearview mirror in your car (yes, I have one). These work best in the summer when the heat of the sun will warm the terra-cotta and the oil so the particles can diffuse. If you wear it around your neck, you can enjoy the benefits of the oil as you move through your day.

- **Bedtime salt bowl method:** Place about ¼ cup of sea salt flakes or Epsom salts in a small bowl. Add 10 to 15 drops of your chosen oil to the salt. Keep it by your bed. The salt slows the evaporation rate of the oils, allowing them to diffuse throughout the night.

- **Ultrasonic diffusing:** This device uses air, water, and ultrasonic vibrations to diffuse the oil. A fine mist is created and released into the air, so it also doubles as a humidifier. This method allows the oil molecules to remain air-bound for several hours. It doesn't affect the structure or therapeutic value of the oil.

- **Electric plug-in diffuser:** These are small units that plug right into an electrical socket. Small absorbent pads, onto which you dot a few drops of oil, are placed inside a heating chamber with ventilation. This allows the aromatic compounds to evaporate into the surrounding air.

- **Car diffuser:** Many companies make car diffusers for their essential oils that just plug into your car's charger outlet. Imagine getting a great smelling, mood-controlling treatment right in the safety of your car as you drive to work or while running errands.

- **Essential oil massage:** Because essential oils are made up of tiny molecules, they pass rapidly through our skin into the bloodstream. The bloodstream quickly and efficiently carries them throughout the body to your cells. Within several hours, they are metabolized and then leave your system. You can massage some essential oils into your body without dilution. Pure essential oils are about 70 times more concentrated than the whole plant, so consult your practitioner about which ones are safe to use directly on skin. You can also dilute essential oils by adding a natural carrier oil. When essential oils can be applied to the skin, they are quickly absorbed into the bloodstream. Some areas of skin—underarms, head, palms, soles of feet—

are more permeable than others. Apply the diluted essential oils to skin areas with gentle massage strokes. Proper topical dilution is: for children aged five and under, 1 teaspoon carrier oil and 2 to 3 drops essential oil; for older children, 1 teaspoon carrier oil and 2 to 3 drops essential oil; for adults, 1 teaspoon carrier oil and 3 to 6 drops essential oil.

- **The foot absorption method:** Before going to bed, massage a few drops of your chosen oils (either "neat" or diluted) into the soles of your feet. They contain some of the largest pores in the body, so the oils are easily absorbed and can reach your bloodstream in just a few minutes.

- **Instead of perfume:** Rather than using store-bought perfumes, you can easily make your own from essential oils. This will have the double effect of causing you to smell good to others and calming you. Combine your favorite essential oils and wear them on your pulse points, behind your ears, on your collarbone, and on both sides of your neck. It is easy to buy amber roller balls online to carry your oil with you wherever you go. It's best to put them in an oil base, but watch that your clothes don't get stained.

- **Spray bottle:** Spraying an essential oil mixture into the air is the easiest, quickest way to change the quality of energy around you. A variety of essential oil mists are on the market or you can make your own. All you need is a glass spray bottle. Fill it with pure or filtered water and add several drops of essential oil. The easy-to-follow guideline: 8 to 10 drops of your favorite essential oils to 8 ounces of water. You can make the mixture more concentrated, though, if you like. Shake it and test it. Experiment and find the right ratio for you. (Or you can purchase a hydrosol, which is not an essential oil, but can also freshen the air.)

- **Compress:** This is a highly effective method for pain relief and emergency first aid. Use a hot compress for relieving chronic pain, muscle aches, or period cramps, and a cold compress for reducing swelling, sprains, and headaches. Put 4 to 6 drops of oil into very hot or icy water. Immerse a folded piece of absorbent material (such as pure cotton or wool) into the water, wring out the excess, and apply to the affected area. Finally, cover the area with a towel or wrap with plastic to keep the cloth either cold or hot. If you are using heat, you can cover the top of the cloth with a water bottle or heating pad.

- **Essential oil bath:** Add your chosen essential oils into a warm bath. This is also a great way to finish off those bottles of essential oils that just have a drop or two left in them. You can also add a few tablespoons of a dispersant, such as Epsom salts or olive oil, which will assist in the absorption of the oils through your skin. Then, just step into the bath and soak. Not only are you absorbing the oils, but you're also inhaling them. A generally safe dose is 5 to 10 drops mixed with ½ to 1 cup of salt or emulsifier. (Please read "As a Precaution . . ." sidebar, page 98.)

⚹ **Sauna therapy:** Add 2 drops of your favorite essential oil to 2 cups of water and place in a sauna. This is a yummy way to get your dose of essential oil calmness.

· · · · · · · · **Can You Ingest Oils?** ·

Unless you're working under the guidance of a certified health prac-titioner, do not take an essential oil internally. You'll need instruc-tion as to which oils are safe, how much to use, and how frequently. You will also spend more money on these oils because they must be made especially for internal use.

· · · · · · · · · · ·⚜· · · · · · · · · · ·

CHOOSING A CARRIER OIL

Most essential oils are not safe to put directly onto your skin, so they are usually di-luted in what is called a carrier oil. Usually, the proportions are 98 percent carrier oil to 2 percent essential oil. Carrier oils come in different sizes, prices, and qualities. The following is a list of the five most commonly used oils. Choose yours based on price and availability:

⚹ **Avocado oil:** The rich, thick, dark green oil derived from the flesh of the avocado is high in essential fatty acids and fat-soluble vitamins, particularly vitamins A, D, and E; potassium; and lecithin. Avocado oil is deeply moisturizing and often rec-ommended for those with sensitive skin. If you're allergic to latex, however, you may also have problems with avocado oil, so it is suggested to do a small skin test before spreading this carrier oil all over your skin. It has excellent skin-penetrating properties that make it perfect to use on dry and flaky skin conditions.

- **Calendula oil:** Calendula oil is an infused herbal oil that is made from marigold flowers. It is an ideal skin-healing oil and can be used for reducing scarring. It is very beneficial for all dry skin conditions.
- **Jojoba oil:** This common carrier oil closely mimics the natural oils in the skin, and is easily absorbed without being greasy. Jojoba oil is not actually an oil as such; rather, it's a form of liquid wax. This makes it more stable than other carrier oils and suitable for use with babies and for those with sensitive skin. It is excellent for use on such skin conditions as psoriasis and eczema. It is also a great treatment for the hair and scalp. Jojoba can be used on its own as a base or in combination with other carrier oils.
- **Olive oil:** This kitchen staple makes for a great carrier oil. To mix with essential oils, it is suggested to use the light version because the extra-virgin has a stronger scent that can overpower the scents of the precious oils.
- **Peach kernel oil:** Peach kernel oil is high in essential fatty acids and contains vitamin E, which makes it wonderful for all skin-healing applications and for use all over the entire body.

········ I'll Have Mine "Neat" ···································

Since dilution can't hurt and can only help, it's a good idea when beginning to use these oils to dilute them, as advised earlier. Most oils should be diluted, but the following can be applied undiluted directly to the skin—or "neat." However, it's still a good idea to patch-test your skin first to make sure you don't get irritated—just dab a drop on your wrist and wait an hour to see whether your skin reacts.

Eucalyptus	Sandalwood
Frankincense	Spearmint
Lavender	Tea tree
Peppermint	Ylang-ylang
Roman chamomile	

············ ⁂ ············

WHO SHOULD AVOID AROMATHERAPY?

Yes, there are some contraindications to be aware of:

- Pregnant women should be careful to avoid certain oils as they may harm the fetus. Speak to your medical practitioner before beginning an aromatherapy program.
- People with severe asthma or a history of allergies should only use essential oils under the guidance of a trained professional and with the full knowledge of their physician.
- People with high blood pressure should avoid stimulating essential oils, such as rosemary and spike lavender.
- People with estrogen-dependent tumors, such as breast or ovarian cancer, should not use oils with estrogen-like compounds, such as fennel, aniseed, sage, and clary sage.
- People receiving chemotherapy should talk to their doctor before trying aromatherapy.
- Rarely, aromatherapy can induce side effects such as rash, asthma, headache, liver, and nerve damage. Stop using the oil immediately if you have symptoms.
- Animal studies suggest that active ingredients in certain essential oils may interact with some medications. Researchers don't know whether the oils have the same effect in humans. Eucalyptus, for example, may cause certain medications, including pentobarbital used for seizures and amphetamine used for narcolepsy and attention-deficit hyperactivity disorder, to be less effective.
- Essential oils are highly volatile and flammable, so they should never be used near an open flame.

ESSENTIAL OILS ARE one way to reach Moodtopia. They will greatly improve your well-being, your overall health, and your sense of connectedness—to yourself, to others, and to this big and amazingly beautiful and generous planet we live on.

PART III

Sara-Chana's Guide to Attaining Moodtopia

CHAPTER SEVEN

FAKING IT

We don't laugh because we're happy; we're happy because we laugh.

—WILLIAM JAMES

A S YOUR LIVER IS BEING SUPPORTED, YOUR BODY IS BEGINNING TO BASK IN adaptogens, and you're incorporating mood herbs and aromatherapy into your life, there are a few inexpensive (and in most cases *free*), easy steps you can take to get your good mood juices flowing. These range from the attitudes you adopt, to the colors you wear, and more. So, let's begin with the simplest Moodtopia technique of all: putting a smile on your face!

BE NICE

There's a story of a Great Rabbi who was wise, caring, and popular because he gave wonderful advice. A woman came into him and said, "I'm a mean person, my mother is a mean person, and even my grandmother is a mean person. What should I do?"

"It's not so complicated," the Great Rabbi answered. "Do nice things."

"What do you mean, do nice things?" the woman shouted at him angrily. "Did you not hear me? I said I'm *not* a nice person."

The Rabbi smiled and calmly replied, "You don't need to be nice or to feel nice to do nice things. Open doors for people, clear someone's plate, smile at a stranger even if you don't feel like it, help a person who's struggling. . . ."

Was the Rabbi teaching this woman to be insincere? Isn't that against everything we've learned? Well, as you'll see in this chapter, science now shows that "faking it"—otherwise known as putting on a happy face—can often create a cascade of positive chemical reactions in our body that will actually help us (and those around us) feel better. It's the next step toward attaining Moodtopia.

Now, I'm not suggesting that you repress what you're feeling. That would be unhealthy. But you can put your negative thoughts on hold for a while and try doing nice things even if you feel yucky. That's not the same thing as repression. And as you'll see in this chapter, faking it, even while you're moody and sad, can help you sort out your negative emotions later.

RANDOM ACTS

Even if you fake it, random acts of kindness make such a difference in your life and the lives of others. Here's one of my all-time favorite experiences that illustrates just this point. I was in my eighth month of pregnancy with my fifth child. Standing a mere five feet tall, I had a belly bigger than a beach ball (and I looked as if I were about to topple over). My cupboard was bare, so I needed to go food shopping. With no babysitter available, I had to bring all my offspring along on this errand. So, there I was, waddling down the street with a double-wide stroller filled with two little kids and my first two hanging on to each side of the carriage running along next to it, making my way to the shops. Suddenly, it started to rain. Now tears began welling up in my eyes. I had one last store to visit to be able to make dinner for these soon-to-be-starving children. The kids began to complain that they wanted to go home, but I needed to do that final bit of shopping.

What had upset me so much in addition to the rain? I was anticipating with a good deal of anxiety how I would get into the store because it was a small mom-and-pop operation and didn't have an automatic door-opener like the supermarket. I was going to have to make a 180-degree turn with the four children and enter the establishment in reverse, pushing the door open with my back. As the rain began to pelt us, I stood in front of the shop, contemplating my dilemma: do I try to go in or not? A young woman literally pushed past me, opened the door, and let it slam in my face. I felt devastated and distraught at her thoughtlessness.

Then, a teenager, maybe sixteen years old, came up behind me, apparently assessed my situation, and said, "Can I help you with the door?" I started crying and laughing at the same time (embarrassing my children once again) and happily, with his assistance, entered the store. I smiled at the young man and said, "Oh my, you're my superhero! Do you have a cape hidden under your jacket?" His one seemingly random act of kindness made me happy beyond belief, and I can tell you that this guy's little gesture took a lot of cortisol out of my body. Even twenty-five years later, it makes me grin to think of it.

So, can one small act of kindness change a life—or even more than one life? Of course it can. Here's what happened after this young man helped me: I was calmer and more patient with my kids. I didn't yell at them in the store. Since I didn't yell at them, they, in turn, didn't fight with one another. Since I was happy, I smiled at them and bought them each a small prize that I promised to give them if they walked back to the house in the rain without complaining. When we got home, they had all cooperated because they wanted to play with their new toys. Because they were calm and happily occupied, I was able to prepare dinner, which meant that by the time my husband came home, not only was there a hot meal on the table, but we were all in a great mood. Wow! And all it took to create this cascade of good feelings was the kindness of one stranger.

If that young man hadn't happened along at that moment, this scenario could have turned out so very differently. Now, I'm not saying that he was excited to help me, or even that he wanted to, but that really wasn't important. All that mattered was that he performed an act of kindness that totally changed my day! When this boy helped me, he also helped himself. Seeing me so happy and receiving my gratitude, he also got a good rush of oxytocin, the "feel-good hormone."

So, the first step in cementing control of your moods is to do random acts of kindness—whether or not you feel like it. Rabbi Manis Friedman, author of The Joy of Intimacy, provides a great example of why your feelings matter less than your kind actions: Imagine that "a poor and hungry person comes to your door. It's really not important to him how you 'feel' or what great advice you have for him. What he needs in the moment is something to eat. And if you give him what he needs, then you have responded appropriately, no matter what you are 'feeling.' Ultimately actions speak louder than feelings."[1]

According to the Random Acts of Kindness Foundation, here's why random acts of kindness are also good for your well-being:

········· **The Benefits of Random Acts of Kindness**[2] ··············

+ **Random acts increase your love hormone.** You don't even have to perform acts of kindness. Simply witnessing them produces oxytocin, the "love hormone," which helps lower blood pressure and improve overall heart health. Oxytocin also boosts self-esteem and optimism.

+ **They increase energy.** About half of the participants in one study reported feeling stronger and more energetic after helping others; many also said they were calmer and less depressed, with increased feelings of self-worth.[3]

+ **Giving to others reduces depression and improves well-being.** This according to Stephen Post of Case Western Reserve University School of Medicine, who serves as president of the Institute for Research on Unlimited Love.[4]

+ **People who volunteer enjoy better health.** Helping others has been shown to protect overall health twice as much as daily baby aspirin protects against heart disease. In another study, people aged 55 and over who volunteered for two or more organizations had an impressive 44 percent lower likelihood of dying early, and that's after sifting out every other contributing factor, such as physical condition, exercise, gender, marital status, and unhealthful habits (e.g., smoking). This is a stronger effect than exercising four times a week or going to church.[5]

+ **Perpetually kind people have 23 percent less cortisol than the average population.**

+ **They also age two times slower.**

+ **They experience less anxiety.** In one study at the University of British Columbia, a group of highly anxious individuals performed at least six acts of kindness a week. After a month, they reported a significant increase in positive moods and relationship satisfaction and a decrease in social avoidance anxiety.[6]

············ ❧ ············

The good news is that kindness can be taught and learned. Mahatma Gandhi said that compassion is a muscle that gets stronger with use. Helen Weng, a researcher at the Center for Investigating Healthy Minds at the Waisman Center of the University of Wisconsin–Madison, has proven this. "It's kind of like weight training . . . we found that people can actually build up their compassion 'muscle' and respond to others' suffering with care and a desire to help."[7] So, go ahead. Make a pact with yourself to perform daily random acts of kindness. If you don't feel it, then fake it. The receiver won't know, and most of the time it won't matter—you'll both feel better for it. Begin with one act a day and see whether you can work up to three. You may not be able to bring about world peace, but you just may prevent a child from getting yelled at, a boss from unfairly firing a worker, or a friend from grousing at her friend—and that friend could be you!

PUT ON THAT HAPPY FACE

Science has shown if you put a smile on your face, even if you're in a lousy mood, your body's neurochemistry will improve. In the nineteenth century, both Charles Darwin and American psychologist William James proposed that facial expressions aren't only the consequence of our emotions, but are actually the cause of them.[8] Today, science has partially proven that our face is directly wired into the emotional centers of our brain. Smiling is a form of facial feedback that elevates our moods.

In the 1960s, James Laird, then a graduate student at the University of Rochester, concocted a ruse. He told a group of students that he wanted to record the activity of their facial muscles under various conditions. He then hooked electrodes to the corners of their mouth, the edges of their jaw, and the space between their eyebrows. The electrode wires plugged into a set of official-looking but nonfunctional gizmos. Next, Laird told the students that he needed them to tense and relax certain muscles. "Now I'd like you to contract these," he'd say, tapping a subject's brows. "Contract them by drawing them together and down." Then, he'd touch the same subject on either side of the jaw: "Now contract these. Contract them by clenching your teeth." Step by step, he'd coax the subject's face into expressions that he wanted—be it a glower or a grin.[9]

In a later, more elaborate version of this experiment, Laird hooked up thirty-two undergrads to fake electrodes, and after tricking them into frowning or smiling, he had them rate cartoons on a scale from 1 to 9, from "not at all funny" to "the funniest cartoon I ever read." When he tallied the numbers, it looked as though the facial feedback had worked: subjects who had put their face into artificial frowns gave the cartoons an average rating of 4.4; those who wore fake smiles judged the same set of cartoons as funnier—the average jumped to 5.5.[10]

Research has shown that the act of forming your mouth into a smile (even if it's a fake one) alters your neurochemistry. Sarah Stevenson wrote in *Psychology Today*, "Each time you smile you throw a little feel-good party in your brain." She explains that smiling activates the release of neuropeptides (molecules that allow neurons to communicate), which work toward fighting off stress. "They facilitate messaging to the whole body when we are happy, sad, angry, depressed, excited. The feel-good neurotransmitters dopamine, endorphins and serotonin are released when a smile flashes across your face as well."[11]

Smiling not only relaxes your body, but can lower your heart rate and blood pressure. As Stevenson explained in *Psychology Today*, "The serotonin release brought on by your smile serves as an anti-depressant/mood lifter. Many of today's pharmaceutical anti-depressants also influence the levels of serotonin in your brain, but with a smile, you don't have to worry about side effects—and you don't need a prescription."[12]

Dr. Christian Jarrett is the author of *Great Myths of the Brain*. He reports in *New York* magazine about a new study led by cognitive neuroscience researcher Dr. Bettina Foster and her team who explored the possibility that when we smile, our expression changes not just our own emotions but also how we perceive other people's emotions. To do this, the team used electroencephalography (EEG) to record the brain waves of twenty-five participants as they looked at photographs of faces that were either smiling or neutral. They focused on two spikes of electrical activity in the brain that typically occur between 150 and 170 milliseconds after observing a face. "These particular spikes are unique to the processing of faces, and are more pronounced when the faces in question have emotional expressions, as compared to neutral ones," Dr. Jarrett explained.[13]

When the participants adopted a neutral facial expression themselves, the team found that these spikes were enhanced after looking at happy faces compared with neutral faces. But what's especially intriguing is that when the participants smiled, "their neural activity was enhanced whether they looked at neutral faces or smiley faces. In other words, *when the participants smiled*, their brain processed or partially processed a neutral face *as if the other person were smiling*."[14]

So, can smiling—even fake smiling—help you control your moods? It's pretty clear that the answer is yes. Even if you're having a horrible day, try smiling through the bad moments. If you walk around all day with a smile on your face, you will bias your mood toward happiness. Not only that, but your smile might spontaneously induce the release of dopamine in someone else's brain—now, that truly demonstrates the power of a smile.[15]

You can learn to fake a smile. Try it. Go into a store and smile at people you pass. Also teach your children to smile. You will be giving them a gift. And, yes, you can tell them that in certain cases it's fine to "fake it." Let's say, you bring your seven-year-old to a retirement home to visit the sick. She may not "feel" like she wants to be nice to people who can look scary. What would your Moodtopia advice be? "Just smile. Even fake it. It will make the older people feel good."

If you're finding it hard to smile, try hanging around children, because they smile far more often than adults do. On average, a child smiles 400 times a day. Happy adults smile 40 to 50 times a day. And the rest of us? We are lucky if we smile 20 times a day. Usually, it's only 7 times a day . . . and grumpy adults manage to crack a smile only once a day.[16]

· · · · · · · · Why Practice Smiling? ·

+ **It makes you seem successful.** Studies have shown that people who smile regularly appear more confident, are more likely to be promoted, and even are more likely to be trusted.

+ **It makes you approachable.** People are more likely to talk to a smiler. They can see that your walls are down, and because you appear open to others, they feel safer.

+ **It works better than chocolate.** Smiling stimulates your brain's reward mechanisms in a way that even chocolate can't match.

+ **It's contagious: People can't help but smile if you smile at them, even if they try not to.** The more you smile, the more others will smile back. Try this with a grumpy friend.

+ **It helps whoever you smile at feel good** (a random act of kindness?).

+ **It releases endorphins and serotonin.** Research has reported that smiling releases these natural pain relievers and antidepressant brain chemicals.

+ **It changes moods.** Even when it's difficult, if you smile when you're feeling blue, it will improve your emotional state.

+ **It lowers blood pressure.** When you smile, there's evidence that your blood pressure can decrease.
+ **It boosts the immune system.** Smiling can actually stimulate your immune response by helping you relax.
+ **It makes you healthier.** Constant smilers seem to have lower stress-hormone levels and a healthier heart.
+ **It makes a lasting impression.** Studies suggest that people are more likely to remember a smiling face.
+ **It builds coping mechanisms.** Someone who smiles a lot tends to be able to handle stress and sudden changes in life. Even if you fake the smile, you will ultimately be able to handle stress better.
+ **It improves work situations.** It's easy to assume that happiness comes from success in work, but that's not quite right. Many studies show that happiness actually comes before job success. It's those people who find reasons to keep smiling that find good results at work.
+ **It builds better relationships.** Smiling helps reduce conflict.
+ **It helps you look younger.** Researchers asked participants to guess the age of strangers in a series of photos. They consistently judged smilers to be younger than they were.
+ **It makes you more appealing.** In studies on attractiveness, smiling faces are consistently rated more appealing. You're putting out a vibe that says you're relaxed, sincere, fun, and attractive. People naturally gravitate toward that.
+ **It's easy.** It takes forty-three muscles to frown but only seventeen to smile.

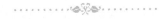

YOU MAKE ME LAUGH!

Want to fake it some more? You need to learn to laugh, even if you don't find something funny, because laughing will help you gain better control of your moods. What? Don't crazy people laugh at nothing?

I once had a client, Michelle, who was having just an awful time of it. She sat on my couch sobbing, black rivulets of mascara running down her face. Through her tears, she said, "If I didn't know this was happening to me, I would think I was watching a comedy." Then suddenly she stopped crying, looked at me, and burst into irrepressible giggles. Guess what? Laughter is contagious, so I also started laughing. We must have guffawed for twenty minutes. We laughed so hard, we doubled over, our sides aching. And more black tears ran down Michelle's face—but this time, they were tears of laughter.

"That was the best thing that has happened to me in the last two years!" Michelle exclaimed after she caught her breath and wiped her eyes. It was then that I realized, in life we can sometimes analyze and analyze and analyze, but what we really need to do for our moods, our body, and our soul is to just laugh.

Laughter is one of the finest, most economical, and easiest Moodtopia measures you can take. It's also one of the best muscle relaxants. It expands blood vessels and sends more blood to the extremities and other muscles all over the body. A good bout of laughter also reduces the levels of stress hormones epinephrine and cortisol. While we're laughing, our mind is without conscious thought processes. All of our senses naturally and effortlessly combine in a moment of harmony, peace, and relaxation.

The week after my laugh-fest with Michelle, I was preparing for a big dinner party in my home. It was an hour before my guests were to arrive, and bedlam had erupted at my house. Music blared from my daughter's room, and the sound of LEGOs crashing to the floor filled the air. "I'll get you this time!" yelled my ten-year-old, as he chased my screaming eight-year-old around their room.

"That's my car!" shrieked the three-year-old, and a tug-of-war ensued as he fought with his six-year-old brother.

"Where is my phone?" complained my daughter as she began turning the living room upside down. "I'm expecting an urgent call . . . ," she moaned, throwing the couch pillows all over the floor.

The kitchen air was alive with the radio newsman describing the latest traffic jam, and the aroma of chicken soup, spicy dips, freshly baked bread, and burning chickens. "Burning chickens!" I screeched as I struggled to my feet from my least graceful hands-and-knees-cleaning-the-bathroom-floor position. Yes, it was confirmed—as three smoking birds were pulled out of the oven—they had indeed burned. But there wasn't any time to mourn my immediate loss.

That's because suddenly I noticed silence, too much silence, and I sensed something was amiss. I ran into the living room to find that my five boys had moved the dining room table up against the wall and had covered the entire living room floor with baby powder.

"Look, Ma, we're ice skating!" My six-year-old's face was beaming as he slid across the floor. Then, my eyes settled on his four accomplices—their faces, hands, black socks, and new black pants were covered with the white powder. They all began "skating" up and down the hall, laughing loudly. The scene: an amalgam of *Swan Lake* and a hockey match.

My heart began pounding. I started to get that feeling in the pit of my stomach. I could tell that I was going to enter my famous "Mom-is-losing-it-again rage." I threw my head back ready to begin my lion's roar, but instead, I walked slowly over to the couch, picked up my baby—who was sticky from raisins despite the bath I'd given her only fifteen minutes earlier—and began to laugh. Slowly at first. Then, the laugh picked up speed and volume, and before I knew it, it was steady and loud.

My children gradually gathered around me, staring in disbelief. "What's *wrong* with her?" my oldest son asked.

"Is she laughing or crying?" my oldest daughter questioned, putting her face very close to mine.

My second son piped up, "I've never seen her like this."

My youngest children began giggling, but my older son wondered, "Should we call an ambulance?"

By this time, I was laughing so hard, tears were flowing from my eyes, and my youngest kids were absorbed in my laughter. "It's okay," I assured my older ones. "This is just an experiment. Instead of yelling, I'm trying to see the humor in our minor catastrophes and laugh when I feel like exploding." I would never laugh if something were really wrong, but our days are filled with difficulties that are not really serious, just distressing. "I'm laughing with you instead of screaming at you," I told them.

The older children looked relieved. Then, they began to chuckle, chortle, giggle, and finally joined the younger children with proper laughter. We all laughed together for about five minutes and then naturally stopped. I looked around at those beautiful faces staring at me. "Okay, kids, we've got forty-five minutes until the guests arrive. I guess I'll just throw some orange juice on the chickens and call it "De Burnt Orange Coq Surprise." My eldest daughter picked up the baby, my older boys began to help me in the kitchen. I asked my younger boys to please begin cleaning up the skating rink, and we all worked as a team.

I knew the dinner party would be great, and meanwhile my children were still laughing rather than feeling sad had I yelled at them.

Faking It

Should we learn to fake laughter? My answer again is—yes! Just like smiling, clinical studies have shown that the body can't tell the difference between "fake" and "real" laughter, and it still reaps the physical and emotional benefits. It's also one of the best ways to ensure you're getting a lot of oxygen. It gives the body an aerobic workout. One pioneer in laughter research, William Fry, claimed it took ten minutes on a rowing machine for his heart rate to reach the level it would after just one minute of hearty laughter.[17] And laughter appears to burn calories, too. Maciej Buchowski, a researcher from Vanderbilt University, conducted a small study in which he measured the number of calories expended in laughing. It turned out that ten to fifteen minutes of laughter burns 10 to 40 calories.[18] In addition, researchers believe that the long series of exhalations that accompany true laughter cause physical exhaustion of the abdominal muscles that, in turn, triggers endorphin release. (This is usually caused by physical activity, such as running or being touched during a massage.)

· · · · · · · · Why Learn to Laugh Even If Nothing Is Funny? · · · · · · · · · · ·

- + **Laughter relaxes the whole body.** A good, hearty laugh relieves physical tension and stress, leaving your muscles relaxed for up to 45 minutes.
- + **Laughter boosts the immune system.** Laughter decreases stress hormones and increases immune cells and infection-fighting antibodies, thus improving resistance to disease.
- + **Laughter triggers the release of endorphins.** The body's natural feel-good chemicals, endorphins promote an overall sense of well-being and can temporarily relieve pain.
- + **Laughter protects the heart.** It improves the function of blood vessels and increases blood flow, which can protect against a heart attack and other cardiovascular disorders.
- + **Laughter burns calories.** Okay, so it's no replacement for going to the gym, but laughing for 10 to 15 minutes a day can burn between 10 and 40 calories—which could be enough to lose 3 or 4 pounds if practiced regularly over the course of a year.
- + **Laughter lightens anger's heavy load.** Nothing diffuses anger and conflict faster than a shared laugh. Looking at the funny side can put

problems into perspective and enable you to move on from confrontations without holding on to bitterness or resentment.

+ **Laughter may even help you live longer.** A study in Norway found that people with a strong sense of humor outlived those who don't laugh as much. The difference was particularly notable for those battling cancer.[19]

. . . . ❧ . . . .

If you're having trouble learning to laugh, hang out with kids and watch them. They laugh with their whole body.

START TAKING CHARGE OF YOUR THOUGHTS

Rabbi Shloma Majeski, the author of *The Chassidic Approach to Joy* and a renowned lecturer on Jewish philosophy, tells us that people are often under the impression that their emotions are beyond their control. Because of this misperception, they resign themselves to negative feelings and moods like sadness or melancholy that seem to take over their lives.

But Rabbi Majeski also teaches us that emotion is born out of the mind. The way we perceive things determines how we feel about them. "Therefore the mind is the key to the heart. We've the ability to control the mind. We can choose what to think about. If we choose not to entertain our minds with depressing thoughts, we won't experience the negative feelings. If we focus with our minds on positive thoughts about our lives and about the future our hearts will feel light and positive."[20]

Rabbi Majeski's philosophy resonates with cognitive-behavioral therapy (CBT), an effective method of resolving clinical depression when accompanied by appropriate medications and/or herbs. CBT is based on the principle that self-defeating, automatic thoughts impact your feelings and vice versa—your feelings impact thoughts. The point of this kind of psychotherapy is to interrupt those self-defeating thoughts—which in turn will put a halt to the negative feelings and help dissipate the depression.[21]

This reminds me of the profound kernel of truth Holocaust survivor Viktor E. Frankl wrote about in his memoir, *Man's Search for Meaning*. "Everything can be taken from a man but one thing: the last of the human freedoms—to choose one's attitude in any given set of circumstances, to choose one's own way."[22] We all have the capacity to choose laughter over tears, smiles over frowns. And sometimes, we can even talk or imagine ourselves out of desperate situations.

When I was in the depths of despair during the most unsettling early weeks of my daughter's ordeal, I visited a therapist for help. I'm usually an optimistic person, but I had gotten stuck in the right side of the Cycle-of-Sanity—frustrated, agitated, angry, sad, and frightened—and could see no way out. The therapist, Dr. Tobi Zausner, who's also the author of *When Walls Become Doorways*, thought that if I learned self-hypnosis, that would help me calm and center myself while our family weathered the crisis. This was a long-term strategy that I could administer to myself whenever I needed it, since no one knew whether or when my daughter's condition would improve or how long we would have to cope with this dire reality. It was a great call.

Tobi asked me to take off my shoes, lie down on her couch, and close my eyes. She instructed me to breathe deeply from my diaphragm so I could relax. Once my breathing became regular, she led me through a guided imagery exercise. First, Tobi told me to visualize in my mind's eye walking down a flight of stairs. She had me go down, and down, and down, and down some more until I entered a lovely outdoor space of my creation. She explained that I loved this space, that I felt safe and secure there—actually it's a real park near my childhood home. I wandered around the park and then lay down on a blanket under an oak tree to rest. This was my "safe place"—somewhere calm and serene where I could go whenever I needed. A place to stimulate my feel-good hormones so I could take better charge of my moods. I stayed there for a while and began luxuriating in a feeling of profound well-being—something I hadn't experienced in weeks. I became less frantic, more grounded. My mind settled. What a blessing.

When we ended our session, as I made my way back up the stairs, I opened my eyes to a new reality. I did have some control of my situation. Even in the glaring lights and cacophony of a hospital setting, I could actually soothe myself.

Was I faking it? In a manner of speaking maybe I was, since nothing had changed in real time. But at least now I had a tool that could help me transform my attitude toward what was happening around me, and that meant the world to me.

It might even work for you.

CHAPTER EIGHT

USING YOUR INTUITIVE SELF TO REACH MOODTOPIA

You must train your intuition—you must trust the small voice inside you which tells you exactly what to say, what to decide.

—INGRID BERGMAN

FOR GENERATIONS, THE TERM *WOMEN'S INTUITION* HAS BEEN USED TO DESCRIBE the unexplainable, nonlogical, sometimes quirky wisdom that women possess. Intuition has been defined as simply knowing something without any reasonable and logical way of knowing it. Dr. Louann Brizendine, the author of *The Female Brain*, refines this definition and narrows it to the female experience: "Women's intuition includes remembering and feeling emotions, heightened senses and sensitivity especially to sound, and the psychic-like ability to understand a situation before it happens."[1]

Do women have such a "sixth sense," or as I tend to call it, an intuitive self? No one quite understands how or why intuition works. But everyone who has ever known a woman will tell you, *yes, it does exist*. After working with so many over the years, I've observed that this trait becomes acute around the teenage years, after a mother gives birth, and then again around perimenopause. As a woman ages, her intuition will render her a "wisewoman." In ancient cultures, such women were honored and revered in their community. Unfortunately, this quality is no longer valued. I've also observed that most girls don't grow up with the understanding that intuition is a gift that blossoms with age. As a result, they don't trust their intuition and spend too much time pushing it away rather than listening to it.

Why is it important to tune into your gut feelings and how does that help you achieve Moodtopia? I believe that connecting with your intuition will help you gain better control of your life situation, which, in turn, will help with your moods. I have heard so many stories in which a woman's intuition came to her rescue. For instance, one of my clients, Emma, gave birth at home. She had a relatively uneventful delivery and her son had great Apgar scores. But the next morning, Emma felt something was not right with her baby and called her midwife. Acting on the midwife's suggestion, Emma immediately ran to her pediatrician. The doctor checked the infant and gave him a clean bill of health. The next day, when the midwife returned, Emma repeated that she felt something was wrong with her child. The midwife suggested a different pediatrician, who also confirmed that the baby was well. By the third day, when Emma was verging on frantic, her midwife took them both to the emergency room.

Fortunately, despite misdiagnoses from two doctors, Emma went with her gut, which told her that something was wrong. At the ER, her son was found to have a heart condition; he underwent emergency surgery. Her instincts were correct, and she had the strength not to be swayed by people who "know more than her." Reflecting on the incident later, Emma told me she had become increasingly frustrated when no one believed her. She snapped at her other children and felt as if she were going to explode. Once the baby received the correct diagnosis—one that confirmed her intuition—Emma felt more stable emotionally, even though it meant that her tiny infant would have to endure cardiac surgery.

Intuition is important in all areas of life, including work. I was recently speaking to my friend Melody, who also confirmed this for me. Melody told me about the twists and turns her medical career had taken her through. "When you complete medical school," she explained, "most interns are not proficient in any one area so they must find their 'match.'" After many placements, she located a position she loved. Her supervisors were great and she enjoyed working with this particular population. One morning, a new manager arrived at the facility. He was said to be a genius who would improve the clinic.

Everyone was excited, but Melody just didn't feel comfortable around this man. Although she loved the work, she felt something was off, so she moved on to another placement. The following year, the government shut down the old facility for fraud. Her former colleagues suffered consequences of the manager's malfeasance. Melody felt bad for them, but she was also happy that she had heeded her intuitive self and avoided what would have been a huge setback in her burgeoning career.

THE COST OF REJECTION

When women go through life denying or minimizing their intuitive thoughts, they often make poor decisions that they know in their gut they could have avoided. They may sincerely feel a certain way, but then, being insecure or ignorant of this wonderful gift, they are easily swayed by their doctors, family members, advertising firms, or peer pressure.

Sadly, ignoring the intuitive self not only hurts you but often your loved ones as well. Everyone ends up feeling disappointed and miserable. Imagine a mom has an initial sense that a certain teacher would be a bad fit for her child. But rather than listening to her inner voice, she accepts the assessment of everyone around her who insist that this teacher is "the best." Yet months later, she wants to pull out her hair because she didn't listen to her own internal warning system. And now her child is suffering.

Or imagine Anita, an up-and-coming manager, meeting Jeff, a new co-worker, who emits a creepy vibe. Since Anita has been programmed to dismiss her first feelings, she talks herself out of her sense of dread and into "liking" Jeff. Then, when he turns on her and blocks her promotion, she says in retrospect with much regret, "I knew I couldn't trust him." Well, why not go with that feeling in the first place?

These situations can be avoided. You need to trust your gut—when something doesn't feel right, it probably isn't. I've experienced that after my clients begin to feel comfortable with me, appreciate this gift, and allow themselves to tune into their gut feelings, they ultimately learn that their intuition is always correct. And when they are honest enough to share with me what their inner voice is telling them, it makes my job as an herbalist and homeopath much easier, as it allows us to come up with quicker and less stressful solutions to their problems.

Judith Orloff, MD, assistant clinical professor of psychiatry at UCLA and author of *Guide to Intuitive Healing: 5 Steps to Physical, Emotional, and Sexual Wellness*, writes, "Women's intuition is a source of great power. The magic comes in awakening it and trusting its guidance in our lives. By learning to trust their intuition, women will come to believe in themselves more strongly and make truly informed decisions."[2]

So, why is it so difficult for us to hold fast to our initial gut feelings, rather than give in to those around us? I believe most of us have spent our life pushing away our intuition so as to be accepted and respected. Is this just a personal challenge or societal programming?

YOUR "SECOND BRAIN": THE BIOLOGICAL ROOTS OF INTUITION

In a study published in the *British Journal of Psychology*, researchers defined intuition as what happens when the brain draws on past experiences and external cues to make a decision—it occurs so quickly, the reaction remains at an unconscious level.[3] But is our intuition formed only by past experiences? And what is this "gut instinct?" Is it just in the hard drive of our brain?

Actually, the age-old terms *gut feeling* and *gut instinct*, which have been used to describe intuitive decisions, are now backed by science. Our "gut" has its own network of nerves called the enteric nervous system (ENS). This is a complex web of about 100 million nerve cells that line the intestines. Sometimes referred to as our "second" brain, the ENS actually develops from the same tissue as our central nervous system (CNS)—the brain and spinal cord—during gestation. That's why the ENS can parallel the brain structurally and chemically.[4]

The neurons in the ENS handle much more than simply digestion, as once thought. Dr. Judith Orloff explains, "Just like the brain, there are neurotransmitters in the gut that can respond to environmental stimuli and emotions in the now." When those neurotransmitters fire, you may get "butterflies" or a feeling of uneasiness in your stomach. Researchers theorize that this "gut response," which sends signals to your brain, plays a large role in intuition.[5] As Adam Hadhazy has written in *Scientific American*, "The little brain in our innards, in connection with the big one in our skulls, partly determines our mental state. . . ."[6]

Dr. Emeran Mayer, author of *The Mind-Gut Connection: How the Hidden Conversation Within Our Bodies Impacts Our Mood, Our Choices, and Our Overall Health*, says, "The system is way too complicated to have evolved only to make sure things move out of your colon."[7] Scientists were shocked to learn that about 90 percent of the fibers in the vagus nerve, the primary visceral nerve, carry information from the gut to the brain and not the other way around.

Scientists describe this gut response as automatic, unconscious thought, whereas reflexive thought requires conscious analysis and takes more effort.

THE FEMALE ADVANTAGE

So, what does this have to do with "women's intuition"? It may have seemed mythical over the millennia, but science has proven women's superiority in this area. Dr. Louann Brizendine writes in *The Female Brain*, "The areas of the brain that track gut feelings are larger and more sensitive in the female brain, according to brain scan studies. Therefore, the relationship between a woman's gut feelings and her intuitive hunches is grounded in biology."[8]

Dr. Brizendine teaches us about girls when they are developing. In a *New York Times* interview she said, "Because of the larger communication center, girls are innately better at reading faces and hearing human vocal tones. Even as a child, all a girl needs to hear is a slight tightening in her mother's voice to know she shouldn't be opening the drawer with the fancy wrapping paper in it. But you will have to restrain the boy physically to keep him from destroying next Christmas's packages. It's not that he's ignoring his mother. He physically cannot hear the same tone of warning."[9]

Sherrie Dillard, author of *Discover Your Authentic Self*, says, "Every day in ways that normally go unnoticed, our intuition works for us. We intuit the unspoken feelings and emotions of our partner, co-workers, children and even the cashier at the grocery store. We know when a loved one in the other part of the house or even miles away is struggling and we can sense the honesty or dishonesty of our children's excuses and the car mechanic's estimate with surprising ease."[10]

HOW TO BUILD YOUR INTUITIVE MUSCLE

It's great that scientists are now beginning to prove that women do have intuitive power, but we need to access it and learn how to fully embrace it.

So, what can we do now? Some of us have retained our naturally biological intuitive self, whereas others seem to have lost it. But I believe with a little retraining, it is possible to reconnect to it. And, if used often and correctly, intuition will grow and become second nature again. Following are a few suggestions that will help make your intuitive self more available to you, so that it will become a trusted friend once more.

Think Like a Spy

I teach my clients to "think like a spy." By that I mean, I want them to have a spy's observational skills. Spies need to be hyperobservant, and they especially need to attend to their awareness because it can often make the difference between life and death. For their own safety, spies are on the alert and have acute visual perception and unbridled hearing. They shut down their babbling thoughts and learn to observe their surroundings. They collect relevant information, which is why their work is referred to as intelligence.

Like a spy, you'll need to develop keen senses through training in how to gather, evaluate, and disseminate vital information. You'll need to cultivate the qualities of paying close attention to detail and compiling and retaining meaningful and relevant data. You need to practice your observational skills and then translate information accurately to tune in to your intuition.

You too must learn to quickly acquire what is called situational awareness (SA), which is a frame of mind in which you are tuned in to your surroundings. You'll also know whom or what to stay away from as well as who could be of help should a problem arise. This exercise will teach you to be in the present moment and not think about the next ten things you want to accomplish. If you learn to do this, you will be able to pick up on the clues your intuition is giving you, so take your time and have fun with it.

Here's how to develop these new skills:

- When you enter a new environment, take a moment to look around.
- Start with the room you're in. Observe it slowly. Notice the color of the walls, the decorations, the smells and lighting. Let everything in the room seep in to your vision. Now, close your eyes. Keep the image of the room in your mind; see it there on the dark screen of the inside of your eyelids. When the vision fades, open your eyes for a few seconds and check the details again. Close your eyes and see it again. Do this several times. Now, with your eyes still closed:
    - Describe the room in as much detail as you can manage.
    - How many blue objects are in the room? What about brown ones? Move from color to color.
    - Now recall all the round objects in the room—flowerpots, vases, teacups. The rectangular ones—the tables, the sofa.

- Ask yourself a series of questions to ignite your observation. Where are the exits? How many windows? What is the layout of the room? How many people are with you? What are they doing?

↠ According to the Personal Safety Training Group, to develop good SA, you need to incorporate into your life a "360 mind-set." "This is a term most often used by the military and law enforcement. It reminds you that our world is not linear. Your observations shouldn't be limited to what goes on in front, to the sides and behind you. Rather, your world is spherical, so become aware of what is happening above you and in some cases below, too."[11]

Listen Intuitively

Really listening to people around you is harder than it sounds because most people are busy thinking about what they want to say next. They haven't been trained to listen with the intent to understand; they have learned to listen with the intent to reply. Take advice from an old saying, "We have two ears and one mouth, so we should listen more than we speak." One of the sincerest forms of respect you can give to your intuitive self and a friend is to actually listen to what he or she has to say. Good listeners don't jump in to complete others' sentences. They don't try to talk over the other person. They are patient and allow a friend to finish a thought so it doesn't get lost or mangled in transit. They wait, so their friend has time and the space to keep going. The most successful people in all areas of life do more listening than talking. Here are some techniques that will help.

↠ **Use the person's name.** People feel honored if you take the time to learn their name. They'll trust you more and it will then be easier for you to read them. If you're not "good" with names, don't be embarrassed that you have to ask a few times. Ultimately, it will make the other person feel you really care about him or her.

↠ **Do more listening than talking.** Listen with curiosity. Speak with honesty. Act with integrity. The greatest communication problem is that we don't listen to understand. We listen to reply. But when we listen with curiosity, we listen for what's behind the words.

↠ **Talk more about the other than yourself.** Remember, you are a spy gathering important information. Allow the other person to give it to you.

- **Face your speaker.** This stance demonstrates your respect and willingness to hear what the person has to say. Look into the other person's eyes—the windows to the soul. To connect to your intuitive self, relax and allow yourself to see beyond the clothes, makeup, and other accoutrements to the "real" person inside.

- **Listen for discrepancies between the words and the tone of voice.** When a conflict occurs between the spoken words and tone of voice, which do you trust? The tone will always take precedence. Become acutely aware of the differences.

- **Remove or minimize distractions.** Distractions are anything that gets in the way of your ability to focus on what the other person is saying. You can't truly listen to anyone while doing something else. That means putting down your phone when you are talking face to face. Distractions make it hard for the person who is speaking to you, but it can make it even more difficult for you to hear your own quiet, intuitive voice. If you want to really receive another person's subliminal messages, make sure you are focused on him or her.

- **Get comfortable with silence.** The trouble with silence is that it makes people uncomfortable. Many feel the need to fill the void with mindless chatter. Don't fear silence . . . honor it! In writing, silence is the space between paragraphs and in stand-up comedy, it's the time it takes for the funny thought to sink in and build. Silence is not a bad thing. It's your ally, and it often occurs when you become receptive. Just as you need a chance to process all the information the other person has said, he or she also needs time to think about what you've said. After all, what's the point of talking if the other person isn't getting it? When we wait in silence, we invite the other person to break it with insights. The individual may feel prompted to expand on a thought, and so you'll learn more.

- **Don't push a person to talk.** Take a seat near him or her and sit quietly. Take a long, deep breath and relax. Come into a receptive, openhearted state and listen. Observe and wait. Spies do a lot of surveillance to gather what they need. Sit patiently and without pressure. In the right time, what needs to be said will be said.

- **Ask open-ended rather than yes/no questions.** Explore your body's reactions further by asking questions to help clarify the source of your feelings. Open-ended questions, such as "How do you feel about that?" or "What makes you say that?" allow the other person to go in any direction and encourage in-depth conversations. The information revealed can help resolve any uncertainties or lingering questions.

- **Be authentically interested.** When you are speaking with others, don't feel as if you need to win them over, don't try to impress them, and don't worry about being judged. Don't be concerned that you may say the wrong thing. Just focus on and listen to what they want to say. This will relieve a lot of tension in your body and will allow you to really find interest in what's being shared.

- **Be sincere in your praise.** The deepest principle in human nature is the craving to be appreciated. *Honest and sincere appreciation* is a most effective tool. When you see a positive attribute, acknowledge it. It will do wonders for you both.

How will this help your intuition? When you become a better listener to others, you will become a better listener to your own quiet voice. Your inner voice never shouts. It never jumps up and down, waving its arms. It never throws a temper tantrum. It simply expects you to attend to it.

Quiet Your Mind

Yeah, right! This may sound easy, but it's not, especially since most of us are multitasking all day. You may have an overactive mind with thoughts that may or may not be correct just repeating themselves in your ear over and over again. Besides, how do you quiet your mind when you're constantly bombarded with external noise: cell phones ringing, e-mails and texts beeping . . . earbuds blasting music directly into your head . . . the television or radio constantly blaring in the background . . . dogs barking . . . construction . . . sirens, cars, trucks, planes, helicopters, jets, and drones— you name it. Then, add the noise of your baby crying, or people on the street laughing or yelling . . . bosses and staff making constant demands . . . loved ones asking you to do this, that, and the other thing for them. The next thing you know, you can't even recognize what quiet means! Your intuition is said to have a "quiet voice," so how can you hear it when it has to compete with all the din that's part of our modern lives?

To become more in tune with your intuitiveness, you'll need to quiet that mental chatter. But how do you even begin to do that? Mediation is the ultimate tool for quieting the mind. It's not so easy and for most it needs to be learned and practiced. For some, meditation is a dream come true. They feel centered, find more clarity, and feel calmer even after ten minutes. For others, however, trying to meditate creates anxiety because they feel they don't know how to do it correctly.

But the goal of meditation isn't to control your thoughts. It's to stop letting them control you (just like our goal in Moodtopia, which is to be in control!). Following are some suggestions that you can easily incorporate into your life. It's what I call your "quick sort-of meditation to center yourself and quiet your mind."

- Buy a set of ear plugs and pop them into your ears.
- Turn off the phone.
- Shut down or move away from your computer.
- Go into a quiet room. If you don't have one, squeeze into a closet and shut the door.
- Take a few moments to tune in and mentally set aside your to-do list.
- You're going to have thoughts. Everyone does. Notice them and just let them go. Visualize them as clouds floating by.
- Sit in silence for at least two minutes. When you are braver, increase it to four minutes.
- That's all there is to it!

Learn to Breathe

Sara-Chana, you may be thinking, what do you mean, "Learn to breathe"? Don't I do it naturally? Of course, we all do. But it's important to breathe properly. Oxygen is the most inexpensive medicine on the planet! At the time of the writing of this book, it was still free, so let's take advantage of it and use it to its fullest.

However, most of us don't take deep soothing breaths from our diaphragm; rather, we take short, shallow breaths that only use the upper part of our lungs. Often, we unconsciously hold our breath just as we hold in our feelings and thoughts. When you hold your breath, you create tightness and muscle spasms around the neck, shoulders, and diaphragm. Your entire chest area can become rigid. Deeper breathing also rids the body of waste products and toxins.

So, how does breathing properly help with being intuitive? When you're stiff, it's harder to tune in to your intuition because muscle pain can dominate your thoughts! But when you take some deep breaths, tension leaves your body, and you're more receptive to zeroing in on your gut. These deep, "cleansing" breaths calm the entire nervous system, allowing you to be more observant of your surrounds and attuned to your inner voice. Here's how:

- Inhale slowly through your nose, then exhale slowly through your nose.
- Or inhale slowly through your nose and then exhale through your mouth, making a loud whooshing sound.
- Practice 2-to-1 breathing (exhalation lasts twice as long as inhalation). If you inhale for a count of 3, exhale more slowly for 6 counts. This technique allows you to concentrate on your breathing.
- Your goal is to fill your diaphragm with air, allowing it to go very deeply into your lungs. In fact, you want to fill up your entire lung area, rather than just your chest. Look at a drawing of human lungs. They are much larger than most people think. Consequently, most of us use only half our lung capacity.
- Think of these deep inhalations as "cleansing breaths," allowing the oxygen to go to the deepest part of your lungs and fill your entire body.
- To relax your jaw, place the tip of your tongue against the roof of your mouth. Keep it there as you practice your breathing.
- Some people imagine inhaling a healing color and then exhaling a color that represents tension and stress. For instance, breathe in a calming light blue and exhale a brown.
- As when quieting your mind, when thoughts come to distract you, picture them as clouds floating in the sky. Then, refocus on your breath.
- You can call this meditation if you want to, but it's ultimately just a wonderful way of stilling your mind, getting oxygen, and healing your body.
- To begin, do this for just two minutes, twice a day. When you get really gutsy, try it for three minutes or more.

Some people find it difficult to make time for breathing. My suggestions: Do it at a red light when you are driving, or while getting a manicure. How about in the shower or after you brush your teeth? Once a day is good, twice a day is better. And wow! What if you could do this four times a day? More deep breathing equals more Moodtopia.

Pay Attention to Your Body's Signals and Learn to Read Others' Nonverbal Cues

Experts explain that nonverbal cues have more than four times the weight of spoken messages—in other words, we're much more likely to pay attention to what an individual does than what she says. For instance, it's entirely possible that someone will say one thing, while that person's body language conveys a completely different message. Say, your assistant is telling you, "Yes, I would love to help you," but her crossed arms and stiff bearing are screaming, "Please don't ask me to do that!"

Also, nonverbal communication is much subtler and more robust. Although the average person may have a vocabulary of 30,000 to 60,000 words, he or she relies on 750,000 nonverbal signals.[12] In fact, scientists have found that we interpret these cues much more quickly and accurately than we do spoken words.[13] Nonverbal communication includes the slightest of movements and facial expressions, such as winking, fake smiles, or slightly raising the eyebrows. See the sidebar "Easily Recognized Nonverbal Cues" for some of the most common signals.

Your body is always communicating with you and giving you signs (say, through your gut responses) that you can either acknowledge or ignore. It always sends out signals to you that indicate your comfort level. But others are also communicating with you nonverbally all the time. To become more intuitive, read your own body's signs while being aware of the messages others send out. Learning about nonverbal communication can help you reach your inner voice. It provides physical cues so that you can pick up on what people around you are really thinking. This helps you gather information more accurately, and can protect you from people who trigger your moods.

· · · · · · · · · **Easily Recognized Nonverbal Cues** · · · · · · · · · · · · · · ·

+ **Arms crossed on the chest:** This can indicate that a person is putting up an unconscious barrier protecting him- or herself from what you're saying. Or it could also mean that the individual is cold!

+ **Eye contact:** In our culture, we are taught from an early age to look into the other person's eyes when speaking. Eye contact can be positive when the overall situation is friendly. It can mean that the other person is thinking deeply about what is being discussed. But it can also mean that the person doesn't trust you enough and "has his or her eye" on you. In a serious or confrontational situation, staring is a sign of hostility and can mean the person is expressing opposition. If, while making direct eye contact, the person is fiddling with something, even while looking at you, it could indicate that his or her attention is elsewhere. If someone is looking straight at you but that gaze is slightly unfocused, this could show boredom.

+ **A harsh or blank facial expression:** The stony face often communicates outright unfriendliness or that one is in command and in control.

+ **Averted gaze, touching an ear, or scratching the chin:** These are all signs of disbelief.

+ **Signals that a person may be lying:** Coughing or clearing one's throat when there's nothing there, a finger to the side of the nose, rubbing one's eyes, blinking too much, speaking loudly, smiling too long, tugging an ear.

Do What You Love as Much as Possible

The feel-good hormone oxytocin was once associated only with having an orgasm or a woman going into labor. But we now know that it can be elicited from many other activities. Studies show that by simply doing what you enjoy, you can activate oxytocin.[14] Why would you want more of this chemical circulating in your body? Oxytocin not only helps you feel good but it also instills trust, increases loyalty, and promotes confidence. It's associated with boosting empathy and reducing anxiety and stress (it lowers cortisol levels). When you're less stressed, it's easier to tune in to your intuitive self and not get caught up in fear that comes from old messages you may have received growing up or from the negative energy of people around you.

If you're in a happier state, you'll be in a better place to hear your often-hidden intuitive voice and to make better decisions. Being open to any creative endeavor seems to positively affect your intuition. Here are some other suggestions that may boost oxytocin in your body.

- Touching and hugging release oxytocin, so hug someone you love. (Hugging is even stronger medicine than touching alone.) No loved ones around? Get a massage. If that's not possible, cuddling works, too—even with your dog or cat.
- Have sex with someone you love!
- Laugh! Read a funny book, watch a comedy, or see a comedian perform.

- Take a walk, in nature preferably (see next section).
- Partake in the arts.
- Call a friend just to chat.
- Being trusted by another person will give you an oxytocin boost.
- Listen to soothing music.
- Give away money to a friend in need. Your friend will benefit immediately, but you may benefit more in the long run.

Spend Time in Nature—Often

We all need to spend time in nature to receive inspiration and grounding; it's just how we're created. So many scientific investigations prove this. For instance, a 2009 study found that the closer someone lives to a green space or park, the healthier that person is likely to be. In fact, those who live closest to a nature preserve or wooded area are less likely to suffer from anxiety or depression.[15] A different study found that people who hike or rest in a forest have a measurably lower cortisol rate, heart rate, and blood pressure.[16] Research at the University of Kansas found that young people who backpacked for three days enjoyed higher creativity and cognitive abilities.[17] People in hospitals who can see a natural landscape get well faster.[18]

I will have much more to say about nature in Chapter 9. But for now, if you can't get into nature, at least bring it into your home. Buy a plant! Even if you don't have a green thumb, such houseplants as philodendrons, rubber trees, spider plants, and most ferns are easy to grow and quite difficult to kill. In Chapter 9, I'll also introduce you to some flowers that are trouble-free and particularly healing to have in the home.

Choose Your Relationships Wisely

If you want to be more intuitive, it's important to keep company with people who are walking a similar path. I always alert my clients who are working toward being less moody that when they undertake this journey toward a mind-set that's deeper and more spiritual, their closest friends and even their family may not accompany them. That's okay, but can be discouraging. This is why it's important to find people with similar aspirations, perhaps in a yoga or painting class. If you can, sign up for a class in the woods or by a beach. It's unlikely the class will be advertised as being "for people looking to tap into their intuitive self," but those who want to better their life, expand their mind, or cultivate their relationship with nature, art, or their physical health will probably gravitate to these kinds of activities. They are the people who won't balk at your desire to become more intuitive.

Your Intuition Is Strongest When the Moon Is Full

The full moon has been honored by cultures all over the world since the beginning of time. In fact, the most important Jewish holidays are celebrated when the moon is full. This is the most spiritual period for the Jewish people as well as many other cultures and religions. Most Hindu holidays fall on the full moon and therefore change from year to year. In fact, in India, the moon (called *Chandra* in Sanskrit) represents the intelligence and intuition of each being and is considered the nourisher of life, the *soma* ("nectar of life"), the Mother within the intuition and intelligence. In Chinese culture, the full moon is honored during the midautumn festival when sons and daughters who have married and left home return to their parents' houses. It's customary to indulge in fragrant moon cakes at that time.

Your intuitive abilities are said to be enhanced during the three days leading to, during, and after the full moon. The moon is connected to the intelligence within the soul, the intuition that is available to the soul, the being, and how it will utilize this intelligence. Next full moon, take time to sit in contemplation of what you have observed and learned this month, this year, even in your lifetime. Make a pact with yourself to open up to your intuition.

Listen to Your Dreams

During the REM stage of sleep, you dream every ninety minutes. Intuition is often considered the language of dreams, since the latter can provide insight into your goals and fears. Or they can be just pieces of your days strung together in strange patterns. But on occasion, they reenact ways you cope with difficult issues in your life. At times, they can compensate for your insecurities. For instance, it's said that dreams in which you're flying pull you out of your rut when low self-esteem is dragging you down.

To become more in touch with your intuition, it may help to keep a dream journal by your bedside. Immediately upon awakening (before getting out of bed), jot down any dreams, images, people, or places you remember. Your thoughts will probably be foggy with many disjointed images, but by keeping a journal you may begin to see a pattern and form some insights. Like exercising a muscle, this dream-recall exercise will strengthen with repetition.

Foster Your Children's Intuition

If given the space, kids are naturally intuitive and can clearly state their feelings. Unlike adults, who often make excuses for what their gut says, kids can provide insight on how intuition works. They quickly determine whether they like or dislike people they meet, and they can usually sense creepy places. However, problems arise when busy adults, who are constantly navigating the many different (and often complex) social events in their lives, ignore their children's instinctual and gut feelings or even dismiss them. Unfortunately, youngsters then walk away with the message that their first intuition is incorrect or unimportant. This is the impression that most of us carry into adulthood.

Begin teaching your children from a young age that what they are feeling and observing is good and safe. That doesn't mean that if your child would rather have ice cream instead of salad, you need to honor this request! But it does mean that if your children feel scared, take the opportunity to talk to them about it, rather than just saying, "Oh, there is nothing to be afraid of." You are still the parent and have adult judgment that is more developed than your children's, but intuitive gut feelings need to be acknowledged and praised. Allow your children to foster their gift of intuition and remind them that they must keep this gift intact as they grow.

·········· How to Support Your Children's Intuitive Self ············

+ Always ask your children how they are feeling, and really listen to their answers.
+ Don't dismiss your child's thoughts out of hand, even if you disagree.
+ If your children say they are scared or uncertain, don't just tell them they shouldn't feel that way; allow them to explain their feelings.
+ Thank your children for sharing their true feelings and tell them how important those feelings are.
+ You don't always have to give in to your children's feelings; just acknowledging them will allow them to continue to develop their intuitive self, be comfortable with it, and allow their gut feelings to have a place in your home so they can gracefully bring them into their adult life.

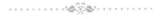

HOW TO TELL THE DIFFERENCE BETWEEN THE INTUITIVE SELF AND THE EGO

As you contemplate connecting to your deepest self, you may react the way many of my clients do. They become nervous when we discuss intuition because they fear they won't be able to distinguish between their inner voices and their ego.

The Voice of the Ego

The ego's main job is physical survival. Through our early years, we often take it on as our predominant voice because it seems to protect us. It is heavily influenced by society, past experiences, culture, and also fear. In fact, although the chief purpose of the ego is protection, more often than not, this voice becomes rooted in our basic anxieties. It likes to talk about wants, security, plans, worries, and stresses. It will push you to achieve more in the hopes that you'll be happier inside, yet that's usually not what happens. It will often also propose the worst possible scenario and be quick to judge and make rash decisions. The ego assumes you live in a world of scarcity. It's a competitive place made up of winners and losers. It will tell you that you can only achieve success if you have more. The ego always likes to be correct, hates being questioned, and loves feeling victimized. Its voice is firm and authoritative, and it communicates with words and emotions that can harm you.

········· How Your Ego May Make You Feel ·······················

> Fearful and anxious
> Jealous
> As if you lack something
> That you are obligated to do something you don't want to do
> That what you feel is wrong or immoral

·············· ❧ ··············

The Voice of Intuition

Your higher self, or intuitive voice, is your soul's internal guidance system. It comes from a bigger place that's not engulfed in fear or unnecessary obligations. In a true sense, it's connected with the universe and something much larger than yourself. It exists to look after you in a different way, to help build you up and not knock you down, to give you the go-ahead to be the best you can be, to allow you to attach to the bigger picture. It won't push you to seek happiness outside yourself, but will keep encouraging you to go inside for answers. The intuitive self believes that there is enough to go around and that everyone deserves to be successful. It doesn't need to compete with the world around you. It guides you to be kind, act real, find happiness in little things, and discover your real talents while you also honor the talents of those around you. Ultimately, it does no harm.

· · · · · · · · · **What You Will Hear from Your Intuitive Voice** · · · · · · · · · · · ·

This feels positive, exciting; it just feels right.
This is moral.
I'm thrilled when I think about it.
I'm hopeful and uplifted.
I feel balance in an unbalanced situation.
I'm at ease; this is simple, uncomplicated.

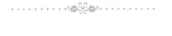

How to Learn the Difference

Be patient with yourself. This will take practice and time. Ego and intuition are the opposites of each other and come from totally different places. Your ego is driven and based on the outer world. It's always seeking approval and security. If you find yourself doing something to impress others or gain attention for what you have, you are acting out of ego. But your intuition is based on love, joy, and finding true happiness in life.

+ **Intuition** guides you to ask someone on a date to share your happiness.
+ **Ego** pushes you to get a date so you won't be alone.
+ **Intuition** guides you to start a business that will help people.

+ **Ego** says you need to start a business to get rich.
+ **Intuition** guides you gently to forgive.
+ **Ego** pushes you to seek revenge.

JUST AS WITH anything else that's important in life, you'll need to work at developing your intuition to feel confident in using it. But it's vital for reaching a state of Moodtopia because it's the basis for so much more, as you'll see in the following chapters.

CHAPTER NINE

FINDING AND CREATING SPACES THAT HELP YOU FEEL GOOD

> At our most elemental, we are not a chemical reaction, but
> an energetic charge. Human beings and all living things are
> a coalescence of energy in a field of energy connected to
> every other thing in the world. This pulsating energy field
> is the central engine of our being and our consciousness,
> the alpha and the omega of our existence.
>
> —LYNNE McTAGGART

WHEN MY HUSBAND AND I FIRST GOT MARRIED, WE LIVED IN MANHAT-tan, where finding an apartment was nearly impossible. We were offered a sublease on a woman's unit while she visited her daughter in Finland. We weren't allowed to alter anything in her place, so we were living in her energy! After about a year, she decided to stay there permanently, so she asked us to please keep her stuff. Some of it was nice, but it wasn't to my taste. Of course, she wasn't permitted to sublet her apartment, and when management found out, they evicted us. Suddenly, we were stuck with her things and no place to live. Since we were newlyweds and didn't have a lot of money, we carried most of her belongings with us as we searched for a new home.

In our next move, we took over an old friend's flat. She kindly sold us her washer and dryer, but also left a lot of her possessions behind. Some of her things were nice, but frankly, some weren't. Still, I didn't have the heart to get rid of her belongings, either. So now, we were living with the old woman's stuff and my friend's old stuff—and nothing of our own. This didn't resonate well with me, but I felt trapped and guilty and foolish for wanting to buy my own furnishings because we were being practical and "saving for our future." In those unsettling days, I had dreams in which I was surrounded by boxes and boxes of things; I sat there amid the clutter, enveloped in other people's energy, not knowing what to do. This environment impaired my ability to control my moods—and I turned into a grouchy bride!

Energy—we don't understand it at all, but everyone feels it. Places and people emit their own vibes. There's an energetic force in the world, just like gravity, and we can use our intuition to attune to or ignore it. When I work with clients, I find that many can't tell me which physical locations make them feel good and which don't. But if you walk into in a certain spot without realizing that you're uneasy, you may leave in a bad mood without understanding why. On the other hand, if you use your intuition to sense where you are and how that place makes you feel, you can be the captain of your energetic yacht rather than susceptible to the turbulence of your emotional tides.

Unfortunately, I learned how important environments are and how they impact us when I lived with my daughter in the hospital. At first, I left the room we were confined to as it was. But the energy in there was horrible and sad. After a week living in gloom, I took action (without the okay of the hospital) and I rearranged what I could to help us both feel better and create the nicest atmosphere and best air flow possible. I brought in fresh flowers and decorated the walls with get-well wishes from my daughter's friends and their kids. I altered the surroundings to boost her (and my) mood.

When seeking to be in control of your emotions, you, too, need to find or create spaces that help you feel comfortable and safe. Yes, it is true certain people will say, "If you're 'balanced,' you should be happy no matter where you are." But that's not necessarily so for everyone. Many of us are subtly affected by the imperceptible energy in our environment in ways we may not be able to explain. I'm sure you'll agree that staying in a five-star hotel overlooking a gorgeous beach will make you feel better than sleeping in a dingy motel next to an abandoned lot filled with rusted-out car bodies and discarded toilets. Unfortunately, not all of us are able to go to that five-star hotel and "chill" when we're having a bad day. So, what to do?

FIRST OF ALL, IDENTIFY AND ATTUNE TO YOUR ENVIRONMENT

Some spaces have "good energy" and some have "bad energy." How do you tell the difference? You can use your think-like-a-spy skills and intuitive capacity to tease out what you sense about where you are. Whether you adventure to new places or simply visit the regular stops along your day, begin to dial in. Step into the space. Pause for a moment and breathe deeply. Before rushing forward, ask yourself the following questions:

- ⌖ "How does this place and/or the people in it make me feel?"
- ⌖ "In my gut, am I comfortable or apprehensive, as if I need to run?"
- ⌖ "Is there something about this spot that makes me happy? Sad? Angry?"

Listen to your intuition to see whether an answer comes to you.

If you discover that you feel uncomfortable in the grocery store you've been shopping at or the gas station you frequent or that café around the corner, it may be worth the extra ten-minute drive or walk to an establishment that has "good energy" for you. Have you been patronizing the business because it's convenient? That may work some of the time, but if you're jittery whenever you're there, the bad vibes in that place could throw you over the edge later. Try other markets, other gas stations, other cafés. This may seem like simple (or very "woo-woo") advice but it can really make a huge difference in your quest to attain Moodtopia.

Those of us who live in open societies can fail to take advantage of our freedoms. Try visiting new *comfort places*—they'll add to your mental health and make you smile. Next month, make time to explore your city or town to find those spots you might never have sought out: that bench behind the courthouse with the rosebush, or the alleyway with wonderful graffiti, or the community garden. Don't feel guilty about spending time identifying the environments that have positive energy and help you feel good. This can improve your mood.

UPEND THE STATUS QUO

Some people live in palaces, some in huts, some in condominiums, some in dorm rooms, and some on farms. Some families have lots of money and hire interior designers to create lavish homes while others squeeze eight people into tiny, cluttered flats. But with awareness and guidance, everyone, no matter what the financial situation, can create a healthy, warm, mood-enhancing environment without spending lots of money. After all, you need to ensure that your home has good energy. This is vital to your health, well-being, and state of mind.

When I first became a lactation consultant, I used to make home visits. Because of my awareness of good and bad energy, I would spend hours cleaning and rearranging my clients' bedroom. I'd say to my clients, "Your bedroom should be your personal oasis and romantic hideaway that encourages relaxation, intimacy, romance, and communication. It must be a nourishing space where people rest, revitalize and reflect." However, I found that many of my clients *survived* in their bedroom, but most were not *thriving* there. They just accepted where the furniture had been placed and which dressers they used. They hadn't bothered to fill their room with colors and pictures they loved. Now, since I also live in Brooklyn where space is limited, I understand this can be a real struggle, but it doesn't mean you have to accept the status quo.

Your bedroom should be a sanctuary of calm. It represents rejuvenation and should only have healing energy in it. When I first began doing home visits, I'd analyze my clients' sleep situation to assess how to make these new mothers' life easier and more nurturing for their own energy as well as their newborn's. I did this even before I'd ask to watch the infant breastfeed. I'd find a cute box or wicker basket and fill it with diapers, wipes, tissues, green clay for diaper rash, and cotton swabs. I'd place this collection of baby goodies on the bed. I'd ask my clients' partner to keep this filled at all times so when the baby cried, Mom wouldn't struggle to find everything she needed for the diaper change. If the family lived in a two-story home, I'd make a box for both floors so everything would be handy.

Next, I'd place a pitcher of water on the night table with some disposable cups, to help the nursing mother stay hydrated. I'd look through the family's linen closet for the prettiest sheets I could find and put them on the bed. I'd ask permission to move lamps around and sometimes even beds. I'd look for a comfortable chair to bring into the bedroom so the new mom could feel at ease while nursing. (Yes, it was a sight to watch me, a five-foot tall woman, schlepping an armchair up the stairs from the living room.) Next, I'd open the windows to air out the place and bring in a live plant. I'd have a bottle of essential oil in my bag and spray it into the air.

I'm a master at getting babies to breastfeed, but what the women thanked me for, more than my skill as a lactation consultant, was the way I made their bedroom better-feeling. I learned that with just a few changes, their moods improved. And once I opened my own office, I made sure that every mom would feel as comfortable as possible in my space.

A SAFE AND HAPPY HOME MAKES FOR BETTER MOODS

When looking for a dwelling, most of us usually find the first available one we can afford and move in without considering anything but the price and possibly the neighborhood and schools. But this was not the case thousands of years ago. In ancient times, when people were given or took over a plot of land, their options were limitless as to where to place the house, its entryways, and the garden. They analyzed the environment to help them make decisions, working within nature to utilize what was available. They needed the front door to bring in air that would cool the home in the summer. But they also had to design a home that didn't capture the wind so it would stay warm in the winter. Since most people grew their own food to sustain themselves, they would decide which area had the best access to water and sunlight in the summer for a garden. They also checked the angle of the moon (which changes, I know) in the evenings to take advantage of as much moonlight as possible.

This practice of environmental analysis developed into the philosophy of feng shui in China over a four-thousand-year period. The term is composed of the Chinese words: feng ("wind") and shui ("water")—the two natural elements that circulate everywhere on our planet. They are also the most basic needs for human survival. Wind—or air—is the breath of life energy, or chi; and water is the liquid of life. Their combined qualities determine our climate, which historically has governed food supply and in turn lifestyle, health, energy, well-being, and ultimately mood.

Initially, people wanted to develop principles that ensured their home—and their tomb—were placed in locations that offered shelter from winter storms, floods, and blazing heat. As the practice of feng shui evolved, the Chinese also started to consider architectural features, such as the placement of fireplaces, windows and doors, mirrors, furniture, and landscaping. Today, architects, city planners, landscape designers, interior decorators, real estate professionals, business executives, and homeowners use feng shui to balance and harmonize home and work environments. The proper placement of design elements is also thought to increase prospects for wealth, health, and improved relationships.

Feng shui is rooted in a holistic view of life, and is not a religion, so it can be incorporated by people of all faiths and backgrounds. All things and creatures are part of a natural order and the energetic flow of chi—the energy force of the world. Our environment is alive, always in flux, ever moving. Everything in this natural order—people, plants, animals, and even inanimate objects such as chairs, pictures, mirrors and beds—is equally alive and swirls with vital energy. The same chi that flows through the world also flows through you. You emit and receive it.

If it's moving properly, chi can make you feel good, but if it's stuck, you can feel bad. Chi can also accumulate in the objects around you. It will stream in through the door and out the windows. The goal of arranging a home in accordance with feng shui is to keep the chi moving "gently" throughout your environment rather than running straight through it or becoming trapped. Feng shui teaches that when energy is stagnant, as would happen with cluttered floors or overflowing closets, or if it moves too quickly through long, dark hallways, or is obstructed with furniture set in the wrong places, this may lead to ill health, domestic strife, mood disorders, or even financial loss.

Jane Morgan, an interior designer and writer, told me that although feng shui appears to be an edgy trend, fit for hipsters and those in the know, its principles have actually been around for centuries and applied by ancient cultures. "The Chinese developed this manual tool for promoting spirituality and well-being at roughly the same time that Biblical Jews appeared to incorporate it into their own holy spaces, including the First Temple in Jerusalem."[1] Amazing!

You, too, can incorporate much of this wisdom into creating a home or workspace that will stabilize your moods. This information is helpful for everyone, no matter what culture or religion. Feng shui philosophy posits that your home is a mirror of what's happening inside you. If it's healthy, then you can be healthy. When a perfect balance is achieved, you may be more successful and less moody. The purpose of incorporating these principles into your life is to align your environment with who you are—to harmonize your energy with your dwelling's energy. It's an art form designed to create a balance in the home which in turn can foster a sense of harmony and Moodtopia within you.

Once you decide that you want to have free-flowing, positive energy, what should you do? Take a walk around your space with a sharp eye. Do you stumble on furniture or rugs? Are wires tangled or getting in your way? Do you have a hard time opening doors? Air should flow around everything; it shouldn't be a struggle for you to get from one room to the next. By making small adjustments, you can help the chi flow freely so that your surroundings support your health, relationships, luck, prosperity, and by extension, your enhanced moods.

Consider what would make your home more pleasant and conducive to good moods and positive energy. Here are some simple, no- or low-cost suggestions, many of which incorporate feng shui ideas. You certainly don't have to do all of them. Choose three to five actions, and see whether they make a difference in your world. If they do, add a few more. And think about which you could easily apply to your workspace:

- **Your front door should be inviting.** As people drive or walk by your dwelling, you want them to be intrigued and feel the good energy. According to feng shui, your front door is the "mouth of chi." This is how energy enters. The amount and quality are determined by the condition of your entryway. If it's open and easy to access, positive energy can enter freely, creating unlimited opportunities and encouraging success, health, harmony, and happiness. So, make your entrance inviting and beautiful. It reflects your desire to receive people, experiences, and opportunities. Use flowers, potted plants (see page 148), a door wreath, banners, or a doormat to provide a warm and friendly invitation.

- **Open your windows more often.** Yes, even in the winter. This allows chi to stream into your home, which, according to the principles of feng shui, can increase free-flowing thoughts and prevent emotional blocks. If you have only a few windows or they open on air shafts, place a couple of air purifiers around the home. Fans also assist in the movement of air/energy.

- **Let the light shine in.** Don't allow a room to remain in darkness during the day—open the shades and curtains. Keeping rooms darkened for long periods (even if you believe you're saving on heating or air-conditioning bills) builds up negative energy. Artificial light can also give you more pizzazz, so now may be the time to replace lightbulbs—the brighter the better. Exchange fluorescent lighting for warm-toned LEDs wherever you can. If your home has dark corners or if you're in an interior apartment, bring in energy with torchière (standing) lamps. They shoot light to the ceiling, which then reflects down into the room and not in your eyes.

Everyone feels better in well-lit environments, but some people truly suffer from being in dark spaces. This is called seasonal affective disorder (SAD). If you get moodier, blue, or even depressed in the winter when the daylight hours are much shorter and gloomy weather blots out the sun, be sure to have enough bright lights in your home. LED lamps are quite intense these days and can provide excellent illumination for pennies a month. If you're particularly troubled by dark days, you can purchase therapeutic lighting especially designed for people with SAD.

Surround yourself with houseplants. They absorb carbon dioxide and give off oxygen and life energy. They help air and energy flow. But be sure to keep only healthy, vibrant specimens. A dead or dying plant is worse than nothing at all! You only want positive energy around you. The Chinese recommend easy-to-grow plants because of what they represent:

- *Lucky bamboo:* This grows quickly and requires very little light or water to survive. The bamboo stem is hollow, which allows free flow of energy, but its exterior is strong. Three to five branches, clustered together, are recommended.

- *The money plant:* You can easily recognize this plant from its braided trunks. It is thought to radiate positive energy and bring good fortune to those who place it in their home or office.

- *Jade plant:* Put one of these succulents at the entrance to your home to welcome guests. Jade is resilient and requires little light or water to remain a vibrant green. Its oval leaves resemble coins and its yellow flowers, stars. It's also considered a good-luck plant and is said to have a calming effect while it attracts material prosperity. It represents deep friendships.

- *Snake plant:* This is a good-luck plant because of its ability to absorb toxins and poisonous gases, such as formaldehyde and benzene. It's among the toughest of all houseplants and can withstand virtually any conditions. In China, the snake plant was treasured because they believed that it bestowed on those who grew them eight virtues: long life, prosperity, intelligence, beauty, art, poetry, health, and strength.

Add flowers to your home. What could be easier or more beautiful? You can use potted, blooming plants but also cut flowers, as long as you discard them when they begin wilting and fading away.

- *Peony:* These sensuous flowers have the most delicate scent. Symbolic of feminine beauty, peonies are used by feng shui practitioners as a love cure.

- **Lotus:** A symbol of perfection, the lotus draws its meaning from the fact that it's untouched by the muddy ponds from which it grows. Chinese medicine uses every part of the plant, so it is a powerful feng shui cure for your home.
- **Tree blossoms:** Branches of blooming trees, such as cherry, apple, dogwood, or peach, bring a sense of newness into your home. Cherry blossoms, in particular, have been used as an aid for romance.
- **Orchid:** In general, orchids have symbolized fertility. Their balance and symmetry are also metaphors for perfection, abundance, spiritual growth, beauty, and purity. No wonder I love them.
- **Narcissus:** The white narcissus is thought to support your career aspirations. It would make a great addition to your work station.
- **Chrysanthemum:** The chrysanthemum symbolizes ease and balance. It is believed to attract good luck as well.

⊁ **Fix what's broken.** Repair broken or malfunctioning objects in your home because they create negative energy. If pipes are leaking, call the plumber as soon as possible! All doors and drawers should open effortlessly. Why be aggravated with little annoyances that can be easily remedied? Make sure your door knobs are tight and working properly. You'll be amazed at what a difference it makes when you literally have a good "handle on things."

⊁ **Observe the rule of pairs.** A friend told me that after a delayed flight, missed connection, and an overbooked hotel, she ended up spending a night in crummy lodgings in Manhattan. It wasn't quite a flophouse, but close. No two things matched in her room—not the headboard with either of the two nightstands (or the nightstands with each other, for that matter), not any of the drawer pulls on the dresser, not the faucets in the sink or shower, not the doorknobs. It was laughable—but it also made her feel edgy . . . and she couldn't wait to get out of there and into her well-appointed room at her chosen hotel.

My friend's reactions were right in line with feng shui wisdom. For the sake of serenity, keep your environment harmonious. Replace mismatched night tables with a set to encourage equality in your relationship. Two identical reading lamps show you want to share your life and home with your loved one. Vases, pictures, throw pillows, and other decor should be displayed in pairs.

⊁ **Declutter.** Recall my funk with the approaching autumn, during which I dreaded that my apartment would be filled with nearly forty coats and jackets. I wasn't too far off. Feng shui principles consider clutter physically, spiritually, and emotionally dangerous. A messy house represents a messy mind—which will affect your work, relationships, and moods. If your space is too full, then opportunities don't have a place to enter. And if there's no room for opportunity in your home, there's no room for opportunity in your life.

One of my herbalist friends told me that the need to gather in every season is innate to women: herbs in spring; fruit and flowers in summer; vegetables in fall; bark and berries in winter. Since we no longer glean our life necessities directly from nature, we now collect *things* that fill our homes—too many pairs of shoes, dresses we'll never wear again, outgrown toys and books, kitchen gadgets, knick-knacks, papers we won't file. Decluttering is one of the most important steps for helping with moods. In her best-selling book *The Life-Changing Magic of Tidying Up: The Japanese Art of Decluttering and Organizing*, cleaning consultant Marie Kondo advises readers to hang on to only the items that continue to give them joy—but to get rid of everything else![2]

➤ **Place your bed correctly.** This is important for harmony and a good night's sleep. If possible, have access to both sides of the bed. Avoid aligning the foot of your bed directly with the doorway. Do your best to position the headboard so there's a solid wall behind it. This creates strong, protective energy around your bed, gives you the ability to have more power while you sleep, and allows you to hold on to your energy. Feng shui philosophy cautions against placing the foot of the bed against a wall as it's believed this can block your career and cause foot and ankle problems. It's also important to see the door while you're in bed, but not have the bed aligned to face the opening. Matching nightstands will create grounding and balanced energy.

➤ **Clear out or organize what's under your bed.** It's tempting to shove junk under the bed, but don't do it. Feng shui experts say that when we sleep, our subconscious is open and absorbs more energy. You don't want negative energy getting stuck under your bed where chi should flow freely. However, if you live in a small space or share a room, this may be impossible to avoid. The most important principle: no clutter under your bed. What to do? Use boxes or closed containers. They should slide in and out easily from under the bed. What you store in the containers should be neat and tidy. Don't keep weapons or sharp metal items, memorabilia from past relationships, or anything needed for work there.

❧ **Check the artwork in your bedroom.** Although many of us do this, feng shui philosophy posits that it's a mistake to display photos of family, friends, or children in the bedroom. Many practitioners believe that it causes your mind to think of others when you should be focused on yourself, your companion, and your rest. Some even believe that pictures of children or relatives may appear to be staring at you and cause anxiety or lack of focus. Consider replacing those photos with calming, soothing images of flowers or nature.

❧ **Limit your use of electronics in the bedroom.** Nowadays, it seems impossible to live without our handhelds—even in bed. When it comes to your moods, though, you need to use them with caution and wisdom so as not to disrupt the energy flow. For instance, it has been shown that the white-and-blue light on the screen can create insomnia because it tells your brain to wake up.[3] Your devices should not be allowed in the bedroom—but if you must use them, put them in a cabinet or behind a closed door before you nod off. One of my clients even eschews TV in her bedroom. "It creates the wrong kind of energy for falling asleep," she told me. Tangled wires can mangle your energy and prevent it from flowing freely—so be sure these are all sorted out neatly.

❧ **Use colors judiciously.** One of my friends painted a small wall in her living room cobalt blue—her favorite color. She perks up every time she passes it. Paint is cheap, and doing one surface (with your landlord's permission, of course), even if it's the interior of the bathroom door, can add a touch of pleasure and a smile to your day. I'll have much more to say about color in Chapter 11, but for now, think about how much fun you'd have with an accent wall that cheers you every time you pass it.

Color can render a room serene, sad, or invigorating. Take time to choose your bedroom's wall color carefully. Consider the energy you want to bring into the room and then pick the hue that will facilitate that. And if you have the freedom to repaint your whole environment, consider which shades will soothe or rejuvenate you. Then go for it!

❧ **Take off your shoes.** Of course, this is a practical way to keep your home clean. If you live in a heavily populated urban area, beware of what you pick up from sidewalks, escalators, and stairways, including everything from animal waste to human bodily fluids. Place a basket or rack for "outside" shoes in a closet near the front door and also a basket of slippers for yourself and guests.

- **Consider the shapes in your home.** According to feng shui philosophy, there are five elements that make up the world: fire, earth, wood, metal, and water. Each one is represented by a shape:

  Fire = triangle

  Earth = square

  Wood = rectangle

  Metal = circle

  Water = wavy

  By including these shapes in your furnishings, you allow the energy of the five elements to flow freely. You can have a round mirror, a rectangular dinner table, a square bowl, a triangular vase, and a painting with wavy lines.

- **Add free-flowing water.** For health, we want movement, so having flowing water around you fights feelings of stagnation. The tinkle of water in fountains represents healthy chi. Consider a water feature in front of your house or a small recirculating fountain on your desk.

- **Use mirrors with a purpose.** Mirrors have an important property: because they reflect light, they also reflect energy. But every mirror must be positioned correctly so as not to reflect negative energy. Placing one at the front door is good, because it prevents negative energy from entering. It is also important to make sure that the image reflected is pretty and positive. If a beautiful bouquet is placed in front of the mirror, then you'll see yourself with the flowers when you pass it. This can make you feel better if you're grumpy or sad. Although many of us do this, it's not recommended to place mirrors in the bedroom, especially facing the bed, as they could disturb sleep.

- **Look for soft edges.** Sharp edges are called *sha chi*—"attacking energy." Feng shui philosophy advises to avoid sharp edges wherever possible. Rounded corners or soft edges on furniture and plants is suggested because they can help increase energy flow.

- **Pay attention to the corners.** When two walls meet to form a corner, feng shui practitioners consider them poison or secret arrows. Ignoring these arrows can cause anxiety in your home. But you can soften these sharp corners by hanging a basket of flowers or wind chimes in the corner or by placing a standing light there.

- **Add rose quartz to your home.** The rose quartz stone is believed to draw love into your life, increase self-love, and heal a broken heart. Buy chunks of rose quartz, rose quartz hearts, or rose quartz lamps, and place them in your bedroom.

- **Burn essential oils, candles, or incense.** This helps increase the fire and air energy in the home, which is both invigorating and calming. Incense and candles have two abilities—one is to diffuse good energy and the other is to purify the air. The careful use of natural candles with essential oils is recommended (see Chapter 6).

- **Pay attention to your bathroom.** When you take a shower, you're removing the bad energy that you may have acquired during the day—a good thing. But the bathroom has the energy of moving water downward and out of your home. In feng shui philosophy, water represents wealth. You don't want to lose your wealth, so it is important to counteract this flow. To balance water energy with wood energy, which is responsible for upward movement and growth, place a live plant or at least a beautiful silk one or photos of trees in the bathroom.

   Be sure to lower the toilet seat lid right after use. This reduces the moisture in the bathroom and limits mold and mildew growth. But even more important, when you flush with the lid up, germs travel six feet in every direction from the bowl.

   Your bathroom should be clean and organized with the flow of chi, but it still is the place where negative energy lives. So no matter how beautifully you have decorated it, the door should remain closed at all times.

FINDING SAFE PLACES IN NATURE

It is hard to achieve Moodtopia if you have elevated cortisol levels and are in a constant state of stress. That's why it is important to see green. Sadly, because my practice is in New York City, I believe most of my clients suffer from "nature-deficit disorder," one of my favorite terms coined by Richard Louv in his book *Last Child in the Woods*. In it, Louv describes what happens to young people who become disconnected from the natural world. He links this lack of nature to some of the most disturbing childhood trends, such as the rise in obesity, attention disorders, and depression.[4]

Unfortunately, more and more, people are cut off from nature. A British survey found that half of the adults polled had played outside at least seven times a week when growing up, whereas only 23 percent of their kids do now.[5] An investigation published in

Nature demonstrated that city living adds to social stress.[6] MRI scans show that greater exposure to urban environments can increase activity in the amygdala, the brain structure involved in such emotions as fear and the release of stress-related hormones. According to this study, the amygdala "has been strongly implicated in anxiety disorders, depression, and other behaviors that are increased in cities, such as violence." The researchers also discovered that people who lived in cities for their first fifteen years of life experienced increased activity in an area of the brain that helps regulate the amygdala.[7] So, if you grew up in the city, you're more likely than those who moved there as an adult to have permanently raised sensitivity to stress.

Indeed, scientific research shows that nature is the place to find serenity and achieve Moodtopia. A short walk in the woods causes measurable improvements in your mood. Stanford's Gregory Bratman designed an experiment in which participants took a fifty-minute walk in either a natural or an urban environment. People who strolled in nature experienced decreased anxiety, brooding, and negative emotion and increased memory performance compared with their urban counterparts.[8]

These changes aren't just emotional. Nature seems to have a healing effect on our physiology as well. For instance, Japanese researchers led by Yoshifumi Miyazaki at Chiba University sent eighty-four subjects to ramble in seven forests, while the same number of volunteers walked around city centers. The forest walkers hit a relaxation jackpot: overall, they showed a 16 percent decrease in cortisol, a 2 percent drop in blood pressure, and a 4 percent drop in heart rate.[9] "A forty- to fifty-minute walk seems to be enough for physiological changes and mood changes," says Kalevi Korpela, a professor of psychology at the University of Tampere.[10] Why is this so? Cognitive psychologist David Strayer hypothesizes that "being in nature allows the prefrontal cortex, the brain's command center, to dial down and rest, like an overused muscle."[11]

PRACTICE FOREST BATHING

So, can being out in a natural setting, even for thirty minutes, help heal your moods? The answer is a resounding yes! In Japan, scientists found people spending time in nature—what they call *shinrin-yoku* (forest bathing)—inhale "beneficial bacteria, plant-derived essential oils and negatively-charged ions" that interact with gut bacteria to strengthen the body's immune system and improve both mental and physical health.[12]

This stress-reduction technique was developed in Japan during the 1980s. Researchers there and in South Korea have found that if you visit a natural area and walk in a relaxed way, your body will calm, restore, and rejuvenate itself. Being enveloped by trees and breathing in their aroma actually helps heal body and mind. If you can't get to a forest, just hanging out by a tree or two can make a difference.

Researchers discovered that the scent molecules of trees are volatile, organic compounds. In 1928, Russian biochemist Boris P. Tokin coined the term phytoncide to refer to a tree's botanical self-defense system. Trees emit various essential oils to shield themselves from germs and insects.[13] Pines and other conifer trees release large amounts of phytoncides to protect themselves. Forest air doesn't just feel cleaner and fresher. Studies have shown that inhaling phytoncides actually helps improve the immune system. When we breathe in these oils, they protect us, too.

· · · · · · · · · **Even Dirt Makes You Happy!** ·

Recent research has determined that soil—yes, what's in your garden—contains a natural antidepressant, *Mycobacterium vaccae*. It has similar effects as antidepressants since it increases the amount of serotonin in the brain. Even cancer patients reported better quality of life with this treatment![14] Maybe that's why people love gardening so much and find it so relaxing! They inhale these bacteria while digging in the dirt.

· · · · · · · · · · · · ·

It's clear that spending time in nature can help you regulate your moods. To begin with, you'll feel calmer and more relaxed, so you won't have to deal with the emotional baggage that comes with city dwelling. And spending time in "big nature," such as hiking in the mountains or gazing at the ocean, provides perspective. It serves to remind us that however serious our problems may seem, they're actually minuscule in the grand order of things.

Indeed, I also believe that observing what often seems like chaos in the natural world is the perfect formula for connecting to yourself and your intuition. It allows you to get a sense of the bigger picture—the wider view. This can help you appreciate that sometimes what looks like a disaster is really a blessing in disguise. This concept reminds me of a story an herbalist once told me. She had just bought a piece of property by the woods. She just loved walking there—no surprise! When an unplanned brushfire erupted, it broke her heart. After it had been put out, the view from her back window was distressing—so many trees destroyed. But soon she noticed that the herb wild lettuce began to grow all over the burnt soil. This is a sedating herb that cools heat in the body and removes pain. She was overjoyed to see this herb healing the land. And she realized how beneficial the fire was and how nature was contributing plants that soothed the land and animals in the area.

Take a look at nature to learn there must be a bigger plan at work that we often can't see when we are caught up in our day-to-day toils, especially in the city. This insight will bring calm and help fuel your intuitive self. Don't forget that trees and plants are here for many reasons, and one of them is to help keep you balanced emotionally and physically.

BEING AWARE OF the influence of environments on your moods and having the courage to make even small adjustments can help you on your path toward Moodtopia.

CHAPTER TEN

CREATING A PROTECTIVE BUBBLE

Certain people can suck the positivity and peacefulness
right out of you. I call these drainers "energy vampires."

—JUDITH ORLOFF, MD, *THE EMPATH'S SURVIVAL GUIDE*

MANY PEOPLE GO THROUGH LIFE FEELING SO VULNERABLE. THEY CAN'T seem to distinguish between themselves and the world around them and are deeply affected by tragedies covered on newscasts, their friends' and neighbors' struggles, and the world's injustices in general. They can be so upset by others' emotions and tragedies that they may find it hard to function. Some of my clients tell me their entire being feels like an open wound into which the world is constantly dropping iodine—ouch. Others describe themselves as a pincushion constantly being stuck. Double ouch! While some women describe their lives in these terms, others say that they're usually fine, but when they're around certain people or in certain situations, they feel at risk and don't know how to protect themselves.

YOUR GUT KNOWS WHAT'S WHAT

As I explained in previous chapters, we all emit and absorb energy from our surroundings and the people in our world. Some of this energy is positive, but some is negative and even destructive. In Chapter 9, we explored how to find and create a protective environment. But what about people? Using your intuition, you can feel in your gut who's safe to be around and who isn't. More often than not, difficult people are sending out vibes that feel toxic to you. So, as you did with your surroundings, you might pause for a moment, breathe deeply, and ask yourself the following questions when encountering someone whom you feel leery about:

- ⇥ "I know what role this person plays in my life, but how does she *really* make me feel?"
- ⇥ "In my gut, am I comfortable or am I apprehensive, as if I need to run? Does he/she feel dangerous to me?"
- ⇥ "Is there something about this person that makes me pessimistic? Frantic? Worn out? Angry? Defensive?"
- ⇥ "How much time do I really need to spend with this person?"
- ⇥ "Do I feel self-conscious and insecure around him or her?"
- ⇥ "Do I feel as if I'm being manipulated?"
- ⇥ "Is this person discounting or disregarding my thoughts or feelings?"
- ⇥ "Is he or she so self-involved, I end up feeling invisible?"

If you find yourself uncomfortable around someone, to preserve your peace of mind, deploy what's called a protective bubble.

ACCESSING YOUR PERSONAL BODY BUBBLE

We may think that we need to imagine an invisible bubble surrounding our body to protect us, but science journalist Sandra Blakeslee, author of *The Body Has a Mind of Its Own*, makes the point that it's already there! "Stand up and reach out your arms, fingers extended. Wave them up, down, and sideways. Make great big circles from over your head down past your thighs. Swing each leg out as far as you can. . . . This invisible volume of space around your body out to arms' length—what neuroscientists call peripersonal space—is part of you . . . Your self does not end where your flesh ends. . . ." You actually have an energy field around you the same way a planet would. Wow![1] That's a novel thought.

Or is it? Of course, we intuitively know about our bubble from daily experience—especially when we feel uncomfortable if someone "invades our space" by standing too near, uninvited. In the TV show *Seinfeld*, the cast joked about these "close-talkers" and how creepy they make us feel. In fact, when jammed together in a crowded place—say, a subway car at rush hour—our inclination is to look up and avoid making eye contact with strangers we may be pressed against, just to preserve a sense of personal integrity. Interestingly, Sandra Blakeslee tells us scientists have discovered that our brain creates maps not only of the inner workings of our body but also of the space or energy field around us.

You can tune in to and activate your own invisible bubble as a protection from other people's energy so that their negativity and what they *say* can't affect you. It will help you immeasurably in attaining Moodtopia. I was first introduced to the concept of using protective bubbles, or energy shields, at one of Dr. Judith Orloff's lectures.[2] "Creating your shield involves visualizing an envelope of white light (or any color you feel imparts power) around your entire body," she explained. "Think of it as a shield that blocks out negativity or physical discomfort but allows what's positive to filter in." Use your bubble to stop another person from draining you of time, energy, peace of mind, emotional calmness, or power. You can create any bubble you want—any color, any texture. Activate it by tuning in to it intuitively or pressing an imaginary button whenever you're feeling threatened. This may sound a little crazy, a bit like a power only superheroes have (indeed, this may truly be a superhero quality), but you have it in you, too.

You can even use this technique in noxious environments in which many people are emitting what you perceive as negative vibes all at once. One of my friends tuned in to her protective bubble at her seven-year-old grandson Joshua's birthday. At his insistence, her daughter and son-in-law held the party at a very loud pizza restaurant filled with arcade games, flashing lights, and lots of screaming, unsupervised children. An introvert, she froze the moment she walked into the establishment. "How am I going to survive three hours in this bedlam?" she wondered. But then she remembered her bubble. She sat quietly on one of the picnic benches, covered herself over with an imaginary blanket of calm, and smiled her way through the party, blocking out as much of the din as she could.

When constructing your protective bubble, keep in mind that you're not being mean to others by diverting their energy. You're simply helping yourself around them so that their funk doesn't affect your mood. Here are some important points to keep in mind:

⇥ No one will notice that you've activated your protective bubble. This is your secret weapon.

⇥ You're not hurting anyone by protecting yourself.

⇥ You can still be kind and gentle to people whose energy you're blocking. You may look them in the eye while they're dumping on you or even screaming. You don't have to ignore them—you just don't have to absorb their energy.

⇥ There's no need to stop liking or even loving the individuals involved. You're only putting an end to the adverse energy they're beaming toward you at this moment.

⇥ You can put up your bubble whenever you need it, even if you're just tired and can't take in another person's life drama right then.

⇥ When you activate your bubble, you're actually giving others a chance to emote and get whatever is bothering them off their chest without its affecting you. This can be a win-win. Venting may be just what these people need, and you can listen and be supportive without shouldering their heavy baggage.

⇥ You can still remain powerful but keep your personal power separate.

WHAT YOU CAN CONTROL AND WHAT YOU CAN'T

The fact is, we really don't have that much control in our lives. When you awaken in the morning, you can't foresee that you'll have a flat tire on the freeway, or that a thunderstorm will knock out all the power in the neighborhood, or that your child will leave school early with the stomach flu. So many things happen outside your capacity to change them. But take heart. One of my favorite sayings is: "We can't control what happens to us in life, but we can control how we respond." You may not have power over these unexpected twists and turns, but you can temper how you react to them.

The same is true with people and *their* energy. You can't control another person's energy. And they can't really *make you* feel sad or angry or uncomfortable. You have the capacity to shield yourself from the negative words and vibe coming at you. You constantly have a secret monologue running in your head. You can decide how you want to feel and how much of other people's energy you want to let in. As Mahatma Gandhi has said, "I will not let anyone walk through my mind with their dirty feet." It may be difficult to create a boundary, especially if a person is close to you, and some may try their darnedest to "get to you," but you can either feel the way *they* want you to, or the way *you* want to. Your mind is really the only place in the world you have that free choice.

Using a protective bubble will guard you from others' negative energy, which in turn can improve your moodiness. Unless you're being physically or emotionally abused, *in which case you must get help and leave immediately,* you can feel safer around someone out to sabotage you or someone who simply wears you down with endless complaints or anxiety.

MAKING YOUR OWN PROTECTIVE BUBBLE

My overwhelmed friend visualized her protection as a blanket—something like a Cloak of Invisibility in the Harry Potter novels or the oft-used "cloaking device" in the *Star Trek* television series. But your bubble can take any shape. Use your imagination! Try seeing it as a dome of white light that surrounds your whole body or as a second layer of skin that hovers a few inches above it. Your bubble can either absorb the pernicious energy or reflect it. If it's the former, just know that the more energy your bubble absorbs, the stronger it becomes. If it's the latter, be a bit more cautious. The energy being reflected can't be targeted, so it might ricochet and hit everything and everyone around you. Still, it's probably the best defense possible.

It may take lots of practice for you to be comfortable with this protective device. And it may take a while to perfect it. But when you're in a stressful situation is *not* the time to begin working on it. Plan ahead. Experiment with conjuring up the imagery when you're calmer and more relaxed, so you can draw upon this resource automatically when you're highly stressed or in the presence of a person who's draining you. If you live in a crowded city or a hectic environment, you can wear this bubble daily or you can activate it only as needed. Here's a step-by-step guide.

· · · · · · · · Create Your Own Protective Bubble ·

+ Before arising in the morning or at night when you lie down to sleep, completely relax your body. Lie as straight as you can and close your eyes. Use the deep-breathing techniques I suggested in Chapter 8 (page 130).
+ If your muscles feel too tight, try a meditation in which you visualize tensing and then releasing each area of your body part by part, moving

from your toes, to your ankles, to your calves... Work your way up to your head. Focus on relaxing.

+ Imagine a bright bubble of golden or white healing light (or any other color you choose) that's as tall and as wide as your body. Envision the bubble settling over you to completely cover you from head to toe, from front to back and side to side. You are now totally inside the bubble and surrounded by its power and protection.

+ The bubble can have a texture, a smell (jasmine, forest pine, the seashore, your mother's chocolate-chip cookies) or anything else you need to feel safe.

+ Slowly take some deep breaths and feel into the safety you've made for yourself.

+ If you believe you've mastered tuning in to your bubble, activate it randomly during the day so you'll have it at the ready when you really need it.

+ Some people buy a necklace or bracelet to remind themselves they have the ability to activate their bubble at will. Many semiprecious stones such as amethyst, lapis lazuli, rose or smoky quartz, and black tourmaline have a history of being protective. You might want to find jewelry inset with these gems for extra security.

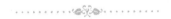

If You're Having Trouble

Attuning to and learning to use your bubble can require time and practice—but it's well worth the trouble, since protecting yourself from others' negative energy is so helpful in developing and maintaining Moodtopia. While you're working at it, you can employ some other tools to help you remain unaffected by others' negative energy.

Use sunlight. If you feel you can't activate your bubble while you're under attack, go to a window. Look in the direction of the sun and feel its healing energy. If it is winter or nighttime, receive the warmth and energy of a lightbulb. Remember the old saying, "It is during our darkest moments that we must focus to see the light."

Fortify yourself. Make sure you're always well rested and well fed. If you're strong in your body, you're better able to resist psychic attacks against your mind and emotions. When you're eating or drinking, say to yourself, "This food (or drink) gives me the strength to protect myself!"

Depend on water. When you're showering or sitting in a bath, allow the water to protect you. Imagine all the negative energy you've received from people washing off you and running down the drain. Let the water encompass your body and help shield it.

Walk away. If you're feeling overwhelmed, don't hesitate to politely excuse yourself. Move out of range of the person's energy. You can be tactful and kind, but if your well-being feels at risk with an individual or in a group, give yourself permission to leave without guilt or explanation. Look for a gush of good energy from other sources. Open the freezer or refrigerator to get a blast of cold. Or stand next to a heater and warm yourself. Imagine that cold air or heat blowing away the negative energy.

Another Point of View

Dutch homeopath Dr. Tinus Smits believed that many of his clients who had trouble placing a self-protective barrier between the world and themselves had their vernix washed off too soon after birth.[3] *Vernix caseosa* is the white, creamy, naturally occurring biofilm covering a fetus's body during the last trimester of pregnancy. This waxy coating protects the newborn's skin and, if not washed away immediately after birth (as is done today in most modern hospital settings), it helps the infant's skin adapt to life outside the uterus during the first week of life.[4]

Vernix is a fascinating substance. It not only has a physiological function but also an emotional and spiritual purpose. Midwives of old used to advise new moms to keep the vernix on their babies for the first few days as they transitioned from living in the world of water to the world of air.

In his homeopathic practice, Dr. Smits found that if he gave his patients who struggled with boundaries tiny doses of the homeopathic remedy vernix, it helped them create an emotional barrier so they could be more functional in the world. In his work entitled *Inspiring Homeopathy*, he taught that since vernix protects the unborn baby during gestation, it was logical that it would protect the patient against outside influences. "The essence of

Vernix caseosa is insufficient separation of its own energy fields from the energy outside," he wrote. "It can easily happen that a person in that state crosses people in the street and picks up the sorrow of somebody who lost his mother, the hate of somebody who is divorcing, the anxiety of somebody who has to face a difficult situation, the hurry from somebody who is late and the nervousness of the whole city."[5]

Often I have also found that when a woman takes a few doses of the homeopathic remedy vernix, it helps her learn to put appropriate boundaries between herself and the world. (Vernix can be ordered from Helios, a homeopathic pharmacy in England [https://www.helios.co.uk/shop/vernix-caseosa] or a pharmacy in Austria [https://www.remedia-homeopathy.com/en/vernix-caseosa/a202582]). But besides this remedy, I also teach my clients how to create an imaginary energetic bubble to protect themselves from the negative energy that constantly swirls around all of us.

INCORPORATING THE BUBBLE INTO YOUR LIFE

One of my clients, Sally, was about to give birth. She was concerned because her mother, Joyce, was coming to help her after her baby was born. Now, many women would welcome their mother's experienced hands, but Sally was frightened. Joyce demanded a lot of attention and made her nervous. She had visited after the birth of her two previous grandbabies, so Sally was reacting from past experience. She had felt so depleted after those interactions, she decided to ask her mom to stay away even though she knew this would crush her.

Before I discussed with Sally the tool of creating her protective bubble, I suggested she start on the homeopathic remedy vernix. Then, we tried an exercise. I asked her to make two columns on a piece of paper. On one side, I wanted her to list all of Joyce's good qualities. The other was to hold an inventory of her more difficult traits. Although the second list was easy, at first Sally struggled to enumerate her mother's positive characteristics. But finally both were completed. Then, I asked her to do the same for herself. We compared the two pages.

Sally was jolted by what she had written. On the "good" column for both of them, she had jotted down: honest, hardworking, caring, willing to help. Sally had always been too busy thinking about how her mother bothered her to consider her positive attributes. What a shock to realize they were very alike in these. For such a long time, she had viewed herself as different from Joyce, so she never considered their similarities. On the negative column, Sally had written that Joyce was a perfectionist, talked too much, and that she was needy and lonely.

Now, I agree that those traits are annoying, but they aren't dangerous. If Sally had written that Joyce was violent, untrustworthy, impulsive, manipulative, destructive, or drunk most of the time, I would have taken notice and even advised Sally to tell her mother to stay away. But I felt we could find a solution that would make my client feel safe while she got the postpartum help from her mother that she needed and that Joyce would cherish.

First, I taught Sally how protective bubbles work and how to access hers. We talked about how she needed to practice connecting to it and using it before the baby's arrival. But then, we went on to a more practical discussion. First, we decided that since Joyce really did want to help and that Sally's other children loved their grandma, we could find ways that Joyce would participate in the arrival of this new family member without pushing Sally's buttons.

To this end, Sally and I made another list. This one set forth tasks her mother could accomplish while she was with the family; these were chores Sally had never thought to ask her mother to do. The first item was sorting through the older children's clothing, collecting items they'd outgrown, and giving them to a charity. Joyce could then organize the clothes that remained and store them neatly in the dresser and closet. Sally knew that her mother would love this activity because she was so into organizing. Next, since the kids were working on their reading skills, Sally decided to buy new books and word games that Joyce could read or play with them while she napped or nursed the baby. She also listed the purchase of tickets for the three of them to go to a theater production she wouldn't be able to attend with the older kids. This would also give her some space.

We jotted down these undertakings so Sally wouldn't have to speak all that much to Joyce. We also made a written schedule, including when Joyce would pick up her grandkids from school. Sally knew that her mother would love the challenge of getting all this done. We kept Joyce so busy in the hopes that she would be exhausted at night and go right to sleep after the kids did—which is exactly what happened.

We took a potentially negative experience, and with preparation and foresight, changed it into a positive one. Sally gave birth to a healthy baby girl and made the decision to not wash off the vernix for the first couple of days of her life. And in the end, Sally was happy that her mother came to stay. Yes, of course, Joyce irritated her from time to time, but Sally's protective bubble helped her through those moments. And she really appreciated the quiet time her mother's presence afforded her, so she could rest and nurture her new infant in peace.

LESSONS TO BE LEARNED

Have you heard the popular expression "I know God will not give me anything I can't handle; I just wish that He didn't trust me so much"? Oh yes, I have felt that myself at times. So, how do we deal with the challenging people in our lives whom we must be around but who also make us unhappy? One of my mentors, Dr. Joel Kreisberg, an integrative medicine physician, helped resolve this conundrum for me. "This difficult person," he explained, "no matter how nasty or bothersome or condemning, is here to teach you a lesson. So, ask yourself, 'What can I learn from this encounter? What wisdom can I glean that will make me a wiser or more patient person?' And appreciate this situation for the wonderful opportunity it really is."

It is said that until we learn our lessons, whatever they may be, we will be tested in life in the same way, over and over again. Dr. Kreisberg works with his patients in what he calls an awareness practice. He prompts them to become observant of what's really going on—to not just blame the other person. He asks that they step back, take a deep breath, and notice whether they or the other person are aggravating the situation. Ask, "What is my impact on other people?" You might begin to notice yourself besides the other person in the situation, and not just react. "Be mindful in the moment," Dr. Kreisberg advised, "and be honest to see if you possibly did something to agitate the other person who is now agitating you."[6]

It could be that your so-called nemesis is truly nasty or mean or impatient or narcissistic, but there is still a lesson in this for you. When Sally compared the lists of her and Joyce's attributes, we had a long discussion about the people she was potentially upsetting. We explored what she could learn from observing her mother's behavior. Afterward, I helped Sally think about her mother with more compassion and kindness, and that led the way to our making Joyce's visit more pleasant for everyone. It also opened Sally's eyes to her own effect on others.

Kabbalah coach Shimona Tzukernik, who created the program The Method, told me, "People are programmed for survival, and depending on their upbringing and experiences, they are trained to respond in different ways. The person upsetting you may not be personally out to get you." That's why one of Shimona's favorite pieces of advice for her clients is, "It's not personal, it is mental."[7] She suggested to see the situation from the other person's point of view—through his or her eyes and not just your own. Shimona told me, "Take *yourself* out of *yourself* and listen completely and silently. Don't let your mind jump ahead and have a comeback line ready before the person finishes his sentence. Stop to see the lesson *you* need to learn." The other person's perspective may appear incorrect from your perception, upbringing, or survival mechanisms, but when you're able to receive another's view, you may also absorb the insight you need to solve the problem.

Shimona went on to say, "In life you're given situations and challenges that are custom-designed for you. It ultimately is for your benefit. If something is difficult, there's a growth opportunity to be found there. Walking away means you will be challenged in that situation again." Growth doesn't come in through the front door and say, "Here I am! I'm your challenge and your opportunity." It comes from where it is least expected—through the windows, pipes, or the chimney. "Pain in life is inevitable," Shimona told me. "But suffering is a choice! Believing that things or people should be a different way brings suffering."[8] As Oprah Winfrey says, "Turn your wounds into wisdom."

So, if you can't change the people or situations around you, for the sake of your moods, you must change your reactions to them and protect yourself.

Now go . . . create your lovely designer bubble.

CHAPTER ELEVEN

REJUVENATING YOUR MOOD WITH COLOR

Mere color, unspoiled by meaning, and unallied with definite form, can speak to the soul in a thousand different ways.

—OSCAR WILDE

FOR YEARS, MY DAUGHTER, WHO IS MY OFFICE MANAGER, AND I WOULD notice that some women seemed "put-together" and emotionally on-their-game even when their lives were challenging or they were in crisis. We observed that there was a certain poise, a finesse and calm to them while others were haggard, overwhelmed, and just out of sorts. But we couldn't put a finger on why. All of my clients were dealing with the rigors of new motherhood. No one was sleeping well. Some had distressed older children constantly tugging at their sleeve for attention. Many suffered with an aching body—and still, one particular group looked fabulous. It didn't make sense. So, we began asking these self-assured women what was behind their glow.

My client Liza is a good case in point. She was in tears, sitting on my couch, holding her parched week-old infant in her arms. Her first baby had been stillborn and this one, her second, a healthy and beautiful girl, was breastfeeding poorly. Liza came to my office to reassure herself that her child was nursing properly, but my scale said differently. When she realized that the child had barely taken in a 0.5 ounce of milk instead of the expected 2.5 ounces, she cried out, "Nothing is going as I planned. My birth was horrible, and now my baby is almost dehydrated." As she looked in the mirror and wiped her eyes, Liza said ironically, "Even though I'm a wreck inside, at least I'm wearing the colors that make me look great." And she did look great . . . dressed in colors that really suited her.

Although Liza had been through a lot and was, understandably, feeling beset, she did look surprisingly wonderful. She was wearing a rust sweater, an evergreen shirt, copper nail polish, gold eye shadow, and she'd applied burnt-orange lipstick to her now quivering lips. Despite her travails and her worried outburst, she seemed as radiant and self-confident as a warm autumn day.

Having your "colors done" was all the rage in the 1980s and '90s. But just because this fad seems passé now—so last century—doesn't mean it's irrelevant to you and your moods today. That's because it really works. Cathy Williams of Seasonal Color Consultation told me that the trend of the '80s has greatly advanced. "Modern color analysis will not put you in a box," she said. "When done right, it harnesses a very large theme (Spring, Summer, Autumn, Winter) and finds its unique expression within the individual."[1]

Color analysis is alive and well today! Many color consultants and fashion stylists (whose jobs include color analysis) work with celebrities, CEOs, lawyers, and others. Some with whom I spoke told me that they advise TV news anchors and personalities about which colors work best on them. Fashion stylist Gwen Marder, who has been dressing on-air talent for twelve years, favors pops of solid, bright colors for her TV clients. "I really like our anchors to wear color because people react in such a visceral way to [it]," Marder said in a *Los Angeles Times* interview. "It's stimulating and pretty to look at on television."[2] According to *Corporate Fashionista*, a style blog for female professionals, executives, and politicians, "Here is the reason it is so important to pay attention to which colors you wear on television! Research tells us that the right color can evoke positive emotions for the task at hand. For a television audience, the screen frames a work of art, so color becomes even more important."[3] But you don't have to be a TV personality to benefit from color analysis.

DO COLORS REALLY MAKE A DIFFERENCE?

Color consultants are people who analyze clients' natural coloring and help them build a repertoire of clothes and accessories that accentuate their attractive features and distract from their less-than-perfect ones. These professionals spend from three to twelve hours and sometimes even longer working to find the hues and tones that bring out the best in a person. They also analyze the shapes and textures of clothing, jewelry, cosmetics, and even the paint on the walls of their clients' home.

How you dress yourself or apply makeup seems so shallow, so trivial—after all, you can't judge a book by its cover, right? Or can you? Color specialist Ginger Burr of Total Image Consultants shared this wonderful story about one of her current clients—a powerful businesswoman. So, you decide:

> After I did a color analysis for a client, she went home and purged her closet of all the colors that did not work for her. For some reason, she decided to keep a yellowy beige dress even though it was nowhere to be found in her palette.
>
> One day, she wore that dress to work. All day, people kept asking her if she was unwell. In the beginning, she reassured them that she was fine and tried to discern why they were posing this question. Finally, after examining herself in the mirror, she realized the color of her dress made her skin appear sallow and lifeless. After the fourth person inquired, she said, "Actually I don't feel all that great," and she went home. Although for a moment she flirted with the idea of keeping the dress and wearing it on days she wanted to escape work early, she feared her boss would eventually catch on. Besides, she liked looking radiant and fresh rather than sickly. So, the dress found a new home, and she became a firm believer in the power of color and the way it affects how a person is perceived.[4]

Call it color therapy, if you want. Do colors make you look healthier or sicker? Do they impact the way others view you? Do they send subconscious messages to people around you? Do they affect how you feel about and carry yourself? You bet they do, and for the sake of Moodtopia, I'm all for resurrecting this trend.

When you can't or shouldn't express your feelings in words, color is a strong non-verbal vehicle. It conveys subliminal messages that others read even before you speak.

+ The colors you wear will impart a healthy glow to your skin and blend with your overall appearance.
+ You will look younger.
+ You will look slimmer.
+ You will look healthier and more well rested.
+ Your eyes will sparkle and shine and dark circles under your eyes will decrease.
+ Overall, your face will appear calmer.
+ The colors will harmonize with your skin tone. It will appear less blotchy and uneven.
+ Your confidence and excitement will be renewed.
+ Your skin will have a healthy, flawless glow. (Okay, you may still need some cover-up.)
+ All of this will help you reach Moodtopia!

MOODS AND COLOR

Color adjectives have been used to describe emotions in dozens of ways: "I feel blue," or "You're black and white to me," or "He was red with rage," or "She was green with envy," or "They were tickled pink," or "It's as if he has a black cloud hovering over his head." These are but a few of the most common color-related expressions. And when we're honest, "our true colors" come shining through, as Cyndi Lauper would say.

Are you in a gray mood today? Or maybe you've been told you have a sunny disposition. According to new research, the colors we use to describe emotions may be more useful than you think. One study found that people with depression or anxiety were more likely to associate their mood with the color gray, whereas happier people preferred yellow. The results, detailed in the journal BMC *Medical Research Methodology*, could help doctors gauge the moods of children or other patients who have trouble communicating verbally. "This is a way of measuring anxiety and depression which gets away from the use of language," study coauthor and gastroenterologist Peter Whorwell of

University Hospital of South Manchester told LiveScience. "What is very interesting is that this might actually be a better way of capturing the patient's mood than questions."[5]

Art, literature, and popular culture throughout history make reference to depression as "blackness" or "grayness." How often do we tell sad people to "brighten up"? Is it true that the world looks bleak when you're depressed? Research has demonstrated that people with depression perceive their vision as less acute and less attuned to visual contrast than when they're not depressed. Science may back up that colors don't seem as bright and that the retinas of depressed patients are less sensitive to contrast during a major depression.[6]

A recent article in the *New York Times* cited research conducted by Andrew Reece at Harvard University and Christopher Danforth at the University of Vermont, which was published in the journal *EPJ Data Science*. The scientists analyzed photos that people post on Instagram and found that they may hold clues to an individual's mental health. "From the colors and faces in their photos to the enhancements they make before posting them, Instagram users with a history of depression seem to present the world differently from their peers," reporter Niraj Chokshi wrote about this investigation. People in this study who were depressed tended to post photos that, pixel by pixel, were bluer, darker, and grayer on average than those posted by people who were not depressed. "We reveal a great deal about our behavior with our activities," the researchers concluded about these findings, "and we're a lot more predictable than we'd like to think."[7]

Even if we don't know exactly how colors affect us in the laboratory, we do know that a lack of color can actually trigger depression, sadness, and moodiness. Take for instance the extreme case Dr. Oliver Sacks described in his book *An Anthropologist on Mars*.[8] His patient, "Mr. I," had been in a minor car accident that resulted in transient amnesia and permanent color blindness. He'd been an artist with a specialty in color. Was he moody? You bet he was. Mr. I was even suicidal.

Unlike someone who was born with genetically based color blindness and who never enjoyed the wide spectrum of hues that most of us perceive, Mr. I was suddenly deprived of a key element in his life and happiness. "It is not just that colors were missing," Dr. Sacks wrote, "but that what he did see was distasteful." Everything looked "dirty" to him, the whites glaring yet discolored, the blacks cavernous—everything wrong, unnatural, stained, and impure. As Dr. Sacks put it, "He could hardly bear the changed appearances of people 'like animated grey statues' any more than he could bear his own appearance in the mirror . . . his wife's flesh, his own flesh, as an abhorrent grey."

Was Mr. I depressed just from the lack of color or his inability to pick up the energy of color? I can't say for sure. But the fact remains that color is a vital part of your existence—one that truly makes a difference in your moods and the way you present yourself to the world. Now's the time to view your life through eyes that absorb color. Take a moment to notice all the hues around you. Don't just stop and *smell* the roses—enjoy their radiance, too. Take your time—colors are candy for your eyes and can lift your spirits. Spend a few minutes every day appreciating the colors around you. Use them wisely, and you've mastered one more step toward Moodtopia.

THE MEANING OF COLORS

It's well known that colors convey specific meanings. For years, advertisers have taken advantage of colors' subliminal power to pitch everything from cars to laundry detergent to hemorrhoid creams!

The marketing industry conducts studies and focus groups nationally and internationally to determine how color affects the decision-making processes. In an article entitled "The Psychology of Colors in Advertising and Marketing," Internet marketing expert Kurt Geer wrote, "If you know it or not, colors speak very loudly to our subconscious and people will have either a positive or negative reaction within 90 seconds." He went on to explain that with people spending most of their days on the Internet, "you have less than 30 seconds to make a good first impression."[9] According to the online publication *Small Business Trends*, "Color can often be the sole reason someone purchases a product, where 93 percent of buyers focus on visual appearance and almost 85 percent claim color to be their primary reason for purchase!"[10] Other researchers have found that up to 90 percent of snap judgments about products are based on color alone.[11]

You, too, can take advantage of the information advertising companies have known and used for years. Colors have subliminal meanings despite the subtleties in one's particular palette. Even though there are hundreds of shades of green and some that would complement you better than others, all shades of it still elicit a general reaction. The broad spectrum of certain colors does communicate specific moods and meanings. Here are some ideas to think about as you plan your wardrobe and decor.

- **Blue** is the most popular color by far. It suggests security, authority, faithfulness, and dignity. People tend to be more productive in blue rooms. This color also promotes rest and calm and can promote deep, relaxing sleep. It can help balance hyperactivity in children, and also encourages imagination and intuitive thinking. For business, it suggests sanctuary and fiscal responsibility.

⇥ **Black** is distinguishing and classic. It suggests authority, power, boldness, and seriousness. It's said to bring protection from external emotional stress. Black can create a barrier between itself and the outside world, providing comfort while protecting one's emotions. It implies self-control and discipline, independence, and a strong will (think of a black belt in karate). But you have to be careful wearing black. It works wonderfully for some people, but for others it can render them intimidating, unfriendly, and unapproachable because of the power the color exudes.

⇥ **Brown** is the color of earth and is abundant in nature. It suggests richness, politeness, helpfulness, effectiveness, genuineness, and reliability. Brown brings to mind feelings of warmth, comfort, and security. It is often described as natural, down to earth, and grounding. In business, brown is perceived as a frugal color—the opposite of frivolity, excess, or waste.

⇥ **Green** is the easiest color on the eye and can improve vision. It suggests health, fertility, freedom, freshness, calmness, healing, tranquility, and (of course) jealousy. It invokes renewal, balance, restoration, and peace—which provide a calming influence and reduce stress. In business, it's used to communicate status and wealth.

⇥ **Gray** is solid, stable, subdued, quiet, and reserved. It can create a sense of calm and composure. It suggests authority, practicality, and earnestness and can provide relief in a chaotic world. Gray does not energize, rejuvenate, or excite. In the business world, it symbolizes tradition and conservatism.

⇥ **Orange** is warm, inviting, and joyful. It suggests pleasure, coolness, excitement, cheer, endurance, strength, and ambition. It invokes feelings of sociability, enjoyable connection, and happiness. It has an emotionally strong presence and promotes extroverted behavior—a fantastic color to use in gathering spaces to encourage interaction and relationship building. In business, it's good for highlighting information on charts and graphs.

⇥ **Pink** creates a feeling of unconditional love, compassion, and understanding and represents giving and receiving nurturing. The mixture of red and white creates a color that tones down the physical passion of red, replacing it with a gentle, loving energy that suggests femininity, tenderness, well-being, and innocence. Pink is romantic, affectionate and intimate, thoughtful and caring. It calms and reassures our emotional energies, alleviating anger, aggression, resentment, abandonment, and neglect. However, you must be aware of pink's feminine qualities and implications in business situations.

- **Purple** suggests spirituality, royalty, luxury, wealth, sophistication, and authority. It's also feminine and romantic. In ancient times, creating purple dyes required a great deal of effort and expense. Because purple is less common in nature, the resources needed to create this dye were much harder and costlier to come by. That's why this color is associated with wealth and royalty. In business, it's upscale and works with artistic types.

- **Red** is associated with high energy and power. It suggests excitement, strength, courage, ambition, sexuality, passion, and vitality. A person wearing red can be seen as aggressive and commanding attention. It's the color our eyes are drawn to first, so a little can go a long way. Red is the most emotionally intense color, stimulating more rapid heartbeat and breathing. It promotes alertness and speed, and connects us to our physical self. In business, it can be associated with debt as well as power.

- **White** can be used to project an absence of color or neutrality. It suggests purity, refinement, devotion, contemporariness, truthfulness, cleanliness, and safety. White space sparks creativity since it can be perceived as a clean state. For business, it can be refreshing. Doctors and nurses wear white to imply sterility.

- **Yellow** enhances concentration, so it's used for legal pads. It suggests warmth, sunshine, cheer, optimism, brightness, mental clarity, and happiness. It promotes creative, clear, upbeat thinking and decision making. It's the most difficult color for the eye to take in, so it can be overpowering if used in excess. Yellow can be helpful in easing depression and encouraging laughter. In business, it appeals to intellectual types and is a good accent color in decorating.

VISITING A COLOR CONSULTANT

A few years ago, after I'd assisted at a birth as a doula, I asked for my customary payment. But my client, Chanie, replied, "My husband refuses to give you a check because he believes you'll only spend it on your children. He wants to buy you a present that would be special to only you." Well! This was a first. I was like, "What?"

And then it arrived: a gift certificate for an appointment with Jessica, a color consultant. Wow! That was *not* what I'd expected! But I loved it even though I was a bit anxious! Black is my basic go-to. What if Jessica told me not to wear it? Nevertheless, I was game and went through the process.

Skin Tone

Color consultants, such as Jessica, first look for skin undertone. Actually, there are two "skin tone" issues: skin overtone (also referred to, confusingly, as skin tone) and skin undertone. The former refers to the superficial color of your complexion—and there are hundreds of variations ranging from very pale, to medium, to mahogany, and all colors in between. Skin overtone can change over one's lifetime due to age and sun exposure, so color analysts don't focus on this very obvious aspect of your outward appearance. Rather, they look at skin undertone—the underlying coloration that is determined by the amount of melanin, or pigment, in the skin. Your undertone doesn't change, ever.

To find your undertone, examine the color of your skin directly behind the shell of your ear or inside your arm, close to your armpit, or between the toes. These areas are less affected by the sun. No matter what the ethnic background—Caucasian, African American, Asian, Latino, Indian, or Native American—one's undertone falls into one of three categories: warm, cool, or neutral.

- If your skin appears yellowish or sallow, you have a warm skin tone.
- If it appears pink, rosy, or bluish-red, then you have a cool skin tone.
- If it appears gray, you probably have an olive complexion with a neutral undertone. The green from your complexion and the yellowish undertone combine to create this effect.
- If there is no cast of yellow, olive, or pink, you have a neutral skin tone.

Observing the veins in your hands and wrists is another way to determine undertone. They will have either a green tinge (a warm skin undertone) or a bluer hue (a cool skin undertone).[12] The vein test works for people of all ethnic origins and has nothing to do with skin color, but results can vary by race: Caucasians tend to have more yellow and red undertones, Black people tend to have more brown undertones, Latinos tend to have more brown and red undertones, and Asians tend to have more brown and yellow undertones.[13]

The Four Seasons

Next, Jessica determined my "season." Season? I was born in February, but what did this have to do with my colors? The season your colors fit into has nothing to do with when you were born or which season you like most. Rather, it's determined by the color scheme that works best for you. Each season has different colors associated with it.

How do we know this? Mostly through the work of Johannes Itten (1888–1967), a Swiss expressionist painter, designer, teacher, and color therapist connected to the Bauhaus school. His theories form the basis of the science and art of color analysis.[14] He was one of the first artists to recognize that colors are energy forces. He called them "radiant energies that affect us positively or negatively, whether we are aware of it or not." Many color experts use an adaptation of Itten's color wheel, which reflects all the colors in nature. His book *The Art of Color* was groundbreaking in its study of how colors impact the viewer. He used psychoanalysis to inform his theories, which set him apart from his contemporaries.[15]

Experiments Itten carried out with his students have also become the basis for color consultants' understanding of the seasons. He asked them to represent the seasons however they wished. He was astonished to find that they each used different colors for the same seasons.[16] But to his greater surprise, despite the wide variation in colors, each student could easily identify which season his or her peers were expressing.[17] "I have never yet found anyone who failed to identify each or any season correctly," Itten wrote. "This convinces me that above individual taste, there is a high judgment in man . . . one which . . . overrules mere sentimental prejudice."[18]

Modern-day color consultants base their analyses on artist Suzanne Caygill's work. In 1942, she originated the concept of color analysis for the individual. After working for years with color and style as a milliner and designer, she had an insight about the relationship between people's natural coloration (as seen in the pigments in their skin, hair, and eyes) and the color harmonies of nature. In addition to color, she also developed her theories on personality and style for each season. While people's color palette is unique to them, Caygill found certain recurring patterns of personality and style, as revealed by the colors.[19]

Suzanne Caygill's breakthrough helps us understand what colors occur naturally during each season. For instance, spring has sharp, vibrant colors that are pure and crisp. Imagine yourself in a field of wildflowers. The sun is becoming more intense, creating wonderful shadows. The summer has relatively muted tones. Think of a hazy, warm day sitting on the sand at the beach, enjoying the sunset. These colors are less vivid than those that occur in spring; they're more hushed and subdued, often melting into one another. Winter has sharper, boldly contrasted colors with lots of grays and blacks. These dark colors are beautifully offset by the white snow. Winter plants include the sharp green of pine trees and deep red berries. Fall is whimsical. Think of the wind swooping up fallen leaves with wonderful dramatic shadows. The season is filled with auburns, burgundies, greens, and browns.

Cathy Williams of Seasonal Color Consultants relies on these concepts when she helps her clients with their colors. She told me that the seasonal designation is a broad category in which countless expressions exist. Nothing is prepackaged. "Think of all the days in all the years in all the centuries of time on the earth. That will give you a good idea of how many versions of Spring, Summer, Autumn, or Winter variations there are." The following is adapted from her website, www.seasonalcolorconsultants.com, where you can find more information.

· · · · · · · · · **What Season Are You?** ·

SUMMER

Summer colors are complex, not easily defined. They're often subdued and luxurious and can include iridescents, jewel tones, floral-inspired pastels, or deep wines and berry tones. Transparent color is especially nice on Summers, who look beautiful wearing colors that are close to each other in value or tone, subtle combinations of blended or related colors (no sharp contrast). Colors worn this way will soothe, center, and empower them. Summers don't feel good in heavy tweeds, anything stiff or thick, or jangly and loud. The key to Summer clothing is femininity. It's soft, graceful, curvaceous, flowing, abundant, rich, and/ or ethereal. Fabrics are soft and romantic: alpaca, angora, cashmere, challis, chiffon, crepe de chine, damask, embossed, faille, jersey, vicuna, Tencel, smooth knits, satin, silk, silk mohair, soft wool, suede, sheer lace, velvet, and velour. Their patterns convey curves, ovals, or figure eights. Think naturalized life forms, birds, wisteria, flowing ribbons, trailing roses, garlands, cascading designs, ferns, watery florals, soft bell shapes, and soft bows.

AUTUMN

Autumn palettes reflect the metallic values of bronze, copper, and ox-idized gold. These colors tend to be rich, mellow, and/or intense with brown undertones, as if toasted. Autumn people can look very attrac-tive using complementary combinations of their particular colors. They might think about Chinese lacquer tones, oriental, Egyptian, and/or Renaissance intensities. When choosing their clothes, they look for lines that are swift or angular (e.g., pockets or epaulets) that suggest power, structure, speed, action, control, and authority. They may also feel great in clothes that feel nubby or have a grounded, earthy qual-ity. They might try tassels, fringe, bangles, scarabs, or feathers, and fabrics such as bark, challis, chenille, damask, Egyptian cotton, faille, linen or flax, gabardine, velvet or velveteen, hand-loomed fabrics, her-ringbone, jersey, burlap, jacquard, lamé, satin, serge, shantung, wool. Autumn patterns include paisley, stripes, plaids, tapestry, leaves, and botanicals and flowers with points. Autumns might also try ethnic, Asian, pagan, or jungle designs.

WINTER

Winter color harmony is focused on white and black, highlighted by pure pigments that have little dilution. The colors are vivid. They elec-trify with deep intensity and are quite striking when worn with neu-trals. Think about stars sparkling like brilliant diamonds in the sky, the delicacy and purity of a snowflake, a tree of leafless branches silhou-etted against a snowdrift, the depth of a silent winter night. In choosing clothing, Winters look for ovals with a classic, smooth, sophisticated feel. They might try garments that are relaxed, with controlled "S" curves. They feel good in well-defined clean lines. Winter fabrics in-clude chiffon, crepe, Swiss cotton, silk jersey, velvet, angora, suede, China silk, gabardine, silk crochet, lace, satin, cashmere, metallic mesh, and fine linen. Winter people aren't attracted to a lot of pattern. If they do wear a print, it might be abstracted in designs that are marbleized, bold, symmetrical, simple, and uncluttered. Winters tend to avoid any-thing fussy, buoyant, or flowery. They don't like a lot of "stuff."

SPRING

Spring colors are clear, undiluted—fresh and joyous to look at. The effect of color on a Spring person is similar: fresh, casual, easy, honest, natural, clear, clean, and refreshing. In choosing clothing, Springs look for circles or anything that suggests roundness or buoyancy: quilted jackets, gathers, ruffles, puffed sleeves, or Peter Pan collars. They might try rounded lace, pom-pom trim, and fun prints in their colors; patterns that convey energy (confetti, polka dots, small checks and plaids), lively florals, or anything whimsical; bows, donuts, lobsters, butterflies, or tacos. Spring fabrics tend to be crisp and fresh-feeling: cotton, crisp lace, crisp wools, dotted swiss, China silk, eyelet embroidery, gingham, organdy, and linen. Springs often feel and look great wearing their versions of red, yellow, and blue together. Colors combined in this way uplift them.

· · · · · · · · · · · · ❧❦❧ · · · · · · · · · · · ·

According to Cathy Williams, "Knowing your season and colors is about having access to your most authentic expression. Your colors, when done correctly, will have you feeling seated, settled, and blessed inside your own skin. In the right colors, your soul ignites."

So, I'm a vibrant Winter! Do I like that medley of colors? Does it make me feel better? That would be an unqualified yes! Now, in the store, I put out my index finger and only stop when I see an appropriate color. It may take me a while to try on clothing, but I need mere minutes to choose *what* to try on.

What am I wearing these days? I have a totally obnoxious, bright orange/red on my list that I *never* would have worn in the past, but when I put on a blouse in that color, strangers stop me all the time to tell me how amazing I look. I have a dazzling purple sweater that takes away all the redness in my face. Black is still my go-to, but now I know to wear it with silver jewelry so I sparkle. Although I've never been drawn to bubblegum pink, I see that I need less makeup if I'm in a pink dress. When I am sad and grumpy, my silky light-blue shirt gives me the boost I need.

+ You'll never buy clothes you won't wear.
+ You'll spend less on makeup.
+ You'll only invest in the items that look absolutely amazing on you.
+ You won't have to guess anymore. You'll know what complements you and what doesn't.
+ You'll save time shopping as you can eliminate 75 percent of colors immediately. (Peek into a store quickly to see whether it has your colors. If not, move on.)
+ All your clothes will match or coordinate with one another, creating more outfit choices from fewer items.

········ ❧ ···········

LETTING GO

Like me, you may feel attached to your own sense of color and style—after all, you've been living with yourself for years or even decades. But your life experience can undermine your ability to be attracted to your best colors. Color consultant Ginger Burr told me, "I am often asked if people are naturally drawn to colors that look good on them. My answer is a resounding . . . sometimes." She put herself up as a perfect example of that. She has red hair. When she was a child, her mother limited her choices because she believed only certain colors look good on a redhead. "So, when I grew up," Ginger explained, "and was able to make my own decisions, I convinced myself that color didn't matter, and I wore whatever I wanted. But I'm sad to admit, it wasn't until someone did my color palette that I really saw the power and impact it had on how I looked!" (By the way, Ginger's mother knew best—the colors she'd chosen for her daughter came up on Ginger's list!)

Your color choices can arise unconsciously from history and social norms—what happens to be in fashion at the moment—and not on what looks best on you. Styles have ebbed and flowed during the twentieth century based on the economic environment. Think of it as an evolution, not a revolution. Technology, politics, and the environment all drive these trends. When the economy is stressed, the fashion industry emphasizes earth tones: burgundies, sage green, burnt orange. These grounded, organic colors help people feel safe. In the '60s, the world exploded in loud, dynamic, and neon colors and dizzying color-on-color psychedelic patterns. The baby boom generation was breaking all norms. Some people were taking LSD, and the unconventional colors and patterns paralleled the experiences they were having. After the madness of the '60s, the colors of the '70s were more subdued. Browns, almonds, and beiges were popular, though they may not have suited everyone's profile.[20]

Personal associations also come into play. If your childhood bedroom was painted lavender, you may gravitate to that hue since it makes you feel safe. Holiday cheer—the red and green of Christmas; the pastels of Easter; the black, red, and green of Kwanzaa; or blue and white of Hanukkah—can also influence how you dress. If a certain color is hip, you may feel driven to wear it so that you can fit in. And, of course, there's always black—great on some people but sepulchral on others. There is a problem with choosing colors that are hip but that don't resonate with you because, as British consultant Candy Gould wrote on her blog, "Wearing the wrong color can drain the face, create shadows under the eyes and have an overall aging effect."[21] And who wants that?

USING YOUR COLORS WISELY

All right, so you've found your true colors. Now you need to know that certain colors are helpful in particular situations. You may find this advice, gleaned from discussions with many color specialists, helpful.

Making a good impression at work: Ginger Burr related another story about how colors can draw people to you or render you invisible. It's not just about what you choose, but also how you combine the colors. She told me about Jenn, a successful speaker and, beyond that, a person with energy and enthusiasm to spare! Together they put together an outfit for one of Jenn's special presentations. "We found her a beautiful purple top and skirt," Ginger explained. "You couldn't take your eyes off her—which is exactly what she wanted."

Next, they looked for shoes to complete the ensemble. Jenn was considering black or nude pumps because they're basic. But Ginger had a different idea. "Since she had wonderful red hair and delicate skin, the black shoes were incongruent with her natural coloring and would have drawn all the focus to her feet. The nude color was okay, but it did nothing to finish the outfit or help Jenn look grounded. Instead, I suggested she consider a pair of bright coral heels. She loved it! 'Finally!' she told me. 'My outward appearance matches my spicy appeal!'"

When you pick which colors to wear from those on your list, be thoughtful about the people with whom you're working. If you're a human resources professional, for instance, who must confront an employee about a sensitive situation, you'll want to put that person at ease. That's the job of your neutral colors—the ones that match some variation of your hair, skin, eyes, and/or the color in your cheeks. These create a harmonious and calming effect. But if you're making a presentation and want all eyes on you, go for your version of the purple ensemble with the coral heels.

Difficult situations: Los Angeles consultant and founder of the company Flying Colors, Inc., Deborah Gordon told me that as she was helping a woman through a divorce, her recommendations changed based on the circumstances. For instance, Deborah advised her client to wear neutral skin-tone colors when she was pleading her case to the judge. These would help her appear truthful and vulnerable. In the middle of the case, enlivening colors that gave an energetic, sparkling look were best. Upon conclusion of the case, Deborah recommended bold colors to show that she was strong, secure, and tough. The client got what she needed from the divorce ruling. She did credit her attorney, but she also felt her colors reinforced her words and gave her the power to stay strong.

Kids: When you take your kids to busy, crowded places, such as shopping malls, amusement parks, or outdoor fairs, the noise and hubbub can be overstimulating. It's best to dress in your neutral skin-tone colors for this outing. They elicit feelings of trust and comfort in others. If you're easy to look at, your child will have a better time refocusing himself—especially if he or she has an attention disorder.

Comparing yourself to your friend: Your coloring may be similar to your pal's, but your personalities may be so different that you each need unique colors to bring out the best in each of you. For instance, two women could have dark hair and light skin and similar palettes, but their choices may still vary widely. One could have a great deal of inner beauty and classy radiance. Her outfits (and especially how she combines colors) would be simple, exuding a soft vibrancy when compared to her friend who is quirky and zesty. The latter can't be too subdued, but she also must balance the brightness of her outfits with her personality—too much, and she'll scare people; too little and she'll surprise them.

Dating: Katherine, one of Ginger Burr's clients, was ready to start dating after a divorce. Ginger told me that Katherine's friends kept nagging her to wear soft, feminine colors. They thought this would make her seem more alluring. But Katherine was dynamic, intense, and passionate. She dressed in black, sophisticated styles. Her raven hair was cut in an edgy 'do, and she wore fairly dramatic makeup. Not surprisingly, she felt uncomfortable with what her friends had suggested. After listening to Katherine, watching her nonverbal communication, and gaining a sense of her personality, Ginger agreed with her client. "Pastels are going to wash you out, and soft, frilly styles will be out of step with your personality. You would feel awkward in those colors and then subconsciously project your distress." Katherine wanted to attract someone she would enjoy and she wanted that person to be drawn to her because he liked who she was and not because she was trying to be liked.

Genuineness is critical to any good relationship. What better time to start expressing yourself authentically than at the very beginning? Katherine was a polished, energetic woman. Although she could wear other colors, she felt comfortable in black *and* it looked good on her.

GOOD VIBRATIONS

Why do colors have such a strong impact on us? Perhaps the answer lies with the physicists and the mystics. One of history's greatest engineers, Nikola Tesla, the man who invented the means to transfer and distribute electricity over long distances (and the namesake of today's self-driving electric cars), once said, "If you want to find the secrets of the universe, think in terms of energy, frequency and vibration."[22]

Every object in the universe vibrates at its own speed. Nothing rests—including our bodies. If the frequency is fast enough, the vibration is emitted as a sound. If it's much faster—by forty octaves—it's emitted as light. In fact, light is vibration.[23] The electromagnetic wave spectrum of visible light produces different colors, which are simply waves vibrating at different frequencies. At one end of the spectrum is red and at the other is violet. Red has the longest wavelength and the lowest frequency, violet has the shortest wavelength and the highest frequency. We sense these waves as color. Visible light is the range of wavelengths within the electromagnetic spectrum that our eyes respond to.

Many people believe that color consultants merely determine which hues make you look better, but Danielle Bryant of Swiss Dot's Color System believes her job encompasses the whole of a person on the inside as well as the outside. "When it comes down to it in quantum terms," she told me, "the colors that work best on you are based on your body's vibration. As quantum physicists have shared, at the heart of everything in this universe is energy. From our bodies to the clothes we wear, it's all made up of energy. With that in mind, I found that when people wear colors that vibrate harmoniously with their body's energy, they feel great. When you wear your colors, your confidence soars, and then your true self shines through."[24]

Deborah Gordon told me that each color has its own energy vibration or temperature. If you find yourself emotionally stressed, you can call upon one of your colors to help calm or empower you—even in creating your protective energy bubble. "Colors can bring out your true natural gifts," she explained to me during a visit to her studio. "We start at the physical, but color helps you look into the invisible. It's the way we emanate energy and vibrate in the world."[25] Color operates on an intuitive level. You can be the best person possible when you stay true to your natural inclinations and soul colors. Color consultant Jessica Riola concurs. "Color vibrates like a person," she told me. "Correct color, and the vibration just clicks."[26]

When colors harmonize with one another, you will look radiant, healthy, and fabulous, and ultimately this can help you attain Moodtopia.

PART IV

Pulling Yourself Together

CHAPTER TWELVE

YOUR 90-DAY PROGRAM FOR BETTER MOODS

ERE'S WHERE YOU PUT IT ALL TOGETHER! THE FOLLOWING IS AN OUTLINE for integrating into your life herbs, aromatherapy, feng shui, colors, and my other suggestions—consider this your hands-on ticket to Moodtopia!

After the 90-Day Program, you'll find a blank Cycle-of-Sanity illustration as well as Moodtopia charts that you can copy into your own journal, along with tips on how to use them. Finally, because our fluctuating energy can wreak havoc on our moods, I've included some of my favorite energy-and-mood-boosting recipes for midday snacks and whenever else you're feeling depleted.

Welcome to Moodtopia!

YOUR 90-DAY MOODTOPIA PROGRAM

It takes about six weeks to develop and sustain a new habit. I've created an easy-to-follow 90-Day Program that incorporates the most salient pieces of the advice I've given in this book. Following this program will not only keep your moods at bay but also help you attain Moodtopia.

The program is divided into four 3-week segments. You might find keeping a Mood-topia journal useful, especially if you're tracking your moods and also your intuitions about who/what/where makes you feel good or crabby. See Chapter 3 and also pages 35–37 for suggestions on charting and journaling. Also, I've included physical exercise here as one of the steps you can take, since there is so much documentation on how it benefits moods.

Bear in mind that if you were a client sitting across from me in my office and you were feeling pretty down, I would be inclined to start you on several healing agents at once—liver support, adaptogens, and mood herbs. However, since most likely you'll be working on your own with this program, I've decided to phase in the various herbal elements so that you will feel comfortable using them. This stepwise approach will also enable you to track your reactions. However, in Chapter 5, I've also offered you the option of trying several mood herbs at once—this is a safe and quicker road to Moodtopia. You can certainly engage in aromatherapy while you're exploring the world of herbal mood remedies. It's all open for you.

WEEKS 1–3

+ Open up to your intuitive self and ask yourself throughout the day how you're really feeling.

+ Start charting your moods in your journal. There are no correct emotions. Just be honest with yourself and become aware of which are most dominant in your life.

+ After years of stress and overwork, you are now going to nourish your liver. Begin by choosing a liver support herb to incorporate into your life two to three times a day.

+ Splurge at your favorite health food store! Buy yourself an essential oil. Many companies make essential oil blends. Take time to find the one you like best—the one that helps you feel most relaxed. Put a few drops on your pillow before you go to sleep. Inhale the fragrance; it will help heal your emotions. Inhale the positive aroma, exhale the bad mood.

+ Pay attention to how smiling makes you feel—and try smiling at the supermarket or at the office, even if you're not particularly happy.

+ Sharpen your observational skills and start thinking like a spy to develop your intuition.

+ Become aware of which environments make you feel good and which don't. Be honest with yourself. And clean up the clutter! See how much better that makes you feel.

+ Set your intention to become more self-aware and self-actualized.

WEEKS 4–6

+ Add an adaptogen to balance your system. Think of your adaptogen as a daily vitamin to refresh your mind and body. Each time you ingest the herb, let it revitalize your whole self.

+ Enjoy your aromatherapy.

+ Make a pact with yourself to perform daily random acts of kindness. Then, do one a day.

+ Sit down and make a list of who makes you feel good and who doesn't. Be honest with yourself. It is important to begin to sense the energy that people emit and not get lost in who you're "supposed" to like or dislike.

+ Start listening to others with curiosity and the intent to understand, rather than with the intent to reply. Pay attention to their nonverbal communications as well as your own.

+ Improve the energy in your home with two feng shui techniques. Choose to rearrange your bedroom or bring in fresh flowers or houseplants.

+ Splurge and work with a color consultant. If this is out of your budget, then find a color you don't usually wear. Buy a new lipstick, nail polish, or scarf in that color to see how it makes you feel. Write about your experience. Do you feel happy? Energized? Calmer?

+ Start to walk daily—even if it is for only fifteen minutes. If you're unable to find that fifteen minutes, park farther away from the entrance to the store or your office. Take the stairs if possible, or just go from sitting to standing a few times at your desk. Concentrate on moving the blood. Stuck blood often means "stuck moods." Allow that circulating blood to push away your moodiness. A wristband activity tracker can help you set and achieve exercise goals.

WEEKS 7–9

+ This is the exciting part! You're at the halfway mark and can now add mood-stabilizing herbs to your liver cleanser and adaptogen. You can begin with one mood modulator or choose up to three that are particular to your personal challenges. Professional herbalists usually use blends that incorporate five to eight herbs that work synergistically. (See Chapter 5.) Eventually, you will be taking about five herbs altogether.

+ Make Cycle-of-Sanity charts and paste them around your house—but especially on your bathroom mirror, where you'll see it at least twice a day.

+ Make sure you're taking your liver herbs and adaptogens daily along with your mood herbs. You can put them into the same small cup and take them all at once.

+ Continue with your aromatherapy.

+ Increase your random acts of kindness to twice a day or more. And keep smiling!

+ Quiet your mind however you can, with earplugs, meditation, deep breathing.

+ Make healthy food choices three times a day to ensure that your blood sugar levels remain stable. Many women become moody simply when they are hungry. Try adding more protein to your diet.

+ Finding an environment that you like or feel safe in is important. Maybe there's a park you always wanted to visit but never had the time. Or check out that new café you noticed in the neighboring town. Search for places where you can throw away your old habits and moods and find fresh spots where your new, "less moody" self can blossom.

+ Add two more feng shui techniques. Perhaps you'll brighten up your entry or simply keep the blinds open during the day.

+ Make sure you're moving every day. Perhaps increase your walks from fifteen minutes to thirty. Spend time in nature as much as possible.

WEEKS 10–12

+ If you find that the mood-stabilizing herbs you started three weeks ago are not decreasing the intensity of your reactions, and your emotions are still overtaking your system, consider experimenting with a different combination of herbs.

+ Make sure that you continue to eat three times a day to keep your blood sugar levels stable.

+ Continue with your aromatherapy.

+ Do what you love to prompt the release of oxytocin. That can mean cuddling!

+ Define the differences between intuition and ego in yourself. Write about it in your journal.

+ Find the time to volunteer or undertake other philanthropic work. Be sure to smile and laugh with your co-workers.

+ Visualize your protective bubble. Practice creating it when you fall asleep at night so you're able to activate it in the morning before you face the day. This way, other people's negative energy can bounce right off you.

+ Buy some new pajamas in your color palette. Also, purchase a shirt that makes you feel happy. Let those new clothes also be your shield against bad energy.

+ Spend a few minutes daily appreciating the colors around you.

+ Consider painting a wall or just a door in your favorite color.

+ If you can, increase your exercise to three to four times a week, and if possible, spend time in nature.

QUICK REFERENCE CHARTS

Use the following chart to help you design your Moodtopia Program. Refer back to the chart in Chapter 5, designating which herb combinations you can use safely.

IF YOU'RE FEELING...

EMOTION	HERBS	ESSENTIAL OILS	ADAPTOGENS
Anxiety/stress	Bacopa, blue vervain, fresh milky oats, holy basil, skullcap, valerian	Cedarwood, clary sage, lemon balm, lemon verbena, sandalwood, vetiver	Ashwagandha, cordyceps, schisandra
Sadness, the blues	Holy basil, lavender, lemon balm, mimosa bark, motherwort, Saint-John's-wort, rose	Bergamot, geranium, grape-fruit, lemon, rose, marjoram, tangerine	Ashwagandha, cordyceps, holy basil, schisandra
Grumpy, short fuse	Chamomile, lemon balm, linden, motherwort, skullcap, valerian	Cedarwood, chamomile, frankincense, geranium, ginger, lemon balm, marjoram, vanilla	Cordyceps, holy basil, schisandra
Brain fog	Asian ginseng, American ginseng, ashwagandha, bacopa, eleuthero, rhodiola, rosemary, schisandra	Eucalyptus, lemongrass, lime, peppermint, rosemary, sage, spearmint	American ginseng, ashwagandha, rhodiola, cordyceps
Burned out, exhausted	Ashwagandha, Asian ginseng, eleuthero, fresh milky oats, rhodiola	Cinnamon, frankincense, ginger, grapefruit, lemon	American ginseng, Asian ginseng, eleuthero, cordyceps, rhodiola
Insomnia	California poppy, chamomile, lemon balm, linden, kava kava, passion flower, valerian, wild lettuce	Lavender, lemon balm, ner-oli, marjoram, sandalwood, vetiver	Cordyceps, holy basil
Lack of Libido	American ginseng, Asian ginseng, ashwagandha, chasteberry, damiana, Siberian ginseng	Cinnamon, ginger, jasmine, lemon verbena, patchouli, sandalwood, rose, ylang-ylang	American ginseng, ashwagandha, Asian ginseng, holy basil

YOU'RE IN IT FOR THE LONG HAUL

Day to day, you may not feel the immediate effects of your Moodtopia journey. You're working subtly with your energy and physiology. However, if you incorporate the remedies that resonate with you, take the long view. Over the course of three months, you'll look back and see that your moods *have* improved. Attaining Moodtopia requires time and patience—and these pay off in the end.

But don't be surprised if you encounter some bumps on your road. You may have a great week, but then fall apart. You may forget to take your herbs. You may backslide and lose it with your kids or co-workers. This is completely natural and normal.

What to do? Don't give up in frustration. Just go back and start again. This is a life journey. Even if you're in a cruddy mood, you can smile at a stranger in the market or wish her "Bless you," when she sneezes. If you hold the door for the person behind you every time you shop, you will start being a nicer, kinder, happier person.

Try the few things that make you feel well again. It may take you five months to reach Moodtopia or it may take two weeks. But however long you need, feel secure in the knowledge that you're on the right road.

Liver Support: A Quick Reference Guide

Since our diet doesn't contain enough bitter plants, most of us can benefit from liver-supporting herbs. Livers that are congested can lead to anger, grumpiness, and depression. Indeed, most livers are congested! The following is a chart of the common physical symptoms that lead herbalists toward the correct liver-supporting herbs.

SYMPTOM	SUGGESTED LIVER HERB
Indigestion	Gentian root, watercress
Skin outbreak, rash, allergies	Burdock root, culver root, milk thistle
Sluggishness	Yellow dock, watercress
Constipation	Dandelion root, culver root, yellow dock
Drinking or partying too much	Milk thistle
Waking and not falling back to sleep	Milk thistle, culver root

The Cycle-of-Sanity

Think of a situation you've been in that you were able to resolve—a fight with your husband, poor grades at school, an argument among your siblings, a social climber at the office. In the chart below, write in what triggered your frustration, anger, and sadness. Then track around to identify your "Aha" moment—the insight that came to you which gave you the energy to solve your problem. Use your own positive experience to remind yourself that you have the internal resources to help you get out of a negative mood and attain Moodtopia. Perhaps think of other incidents. The more you reinforce your own capacity to resolve issues, the more confident you'll feel going forward.

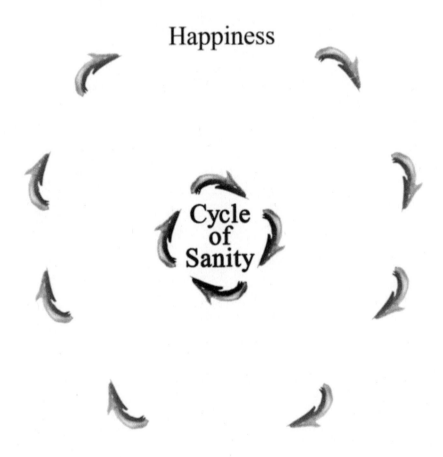

Happiness

Cycle
of
Sanity

Charting Your Moods

In Chapter 3, we talked about charting your moods. Here are some tips for making and using your own Moodtopia chart:

- Decide on the format you want to use.
- Choose what you will be tracking. Mood charts can be as simple or elaborate as you make them. You may wish to follow one to two moods a week—or all of them. It's totally up to you.
- What to write down: You can simply list a few descriptive words or score your moods on a scale of 1 to 10.
- Note anything significant that may have affected your mood: This could include weather changes, sleeping partners, excess urination at night, an argument, hunger, alcohol, a cold, your menstrual cycle, a disturbing person or place. You are looking for patterns that can be personal triggers for you.
- Determine how many times a day you would like to make entries in your chart. If you are awake for 18 hours a day, it might be most helpful to chart 3 times a day—every 6 hours. Or you might make entries whenever your mood shifts.

Copy and use the following calendar to note when and where you feel grumpy.

My Moodtopia Chart							
Week: 1							
	Mon	Tue	Wed	Thu	Fri	Sat	Sun
7:00 AM							
8:00 AM							
9:00 AM							
10:00 AM							
11:00 AM							
Noon							
1:00 PM							
2:00 PM							
3:00 PM							
4:00 PM							
5:00 PM							
6:00 PM							
7:00 PM							
8:00 PM							
9:00 PM							
10:00 PM							

MOOD-BOOSTING RECIPES

As far back as the 1980s, Drs. Richard and Judith Wurtman at the Massachusetts Institute of Technology proposed that carbs increase serotonin and tryptophan—depression-fighting neurochemicals—in the brain.[1] It has also been speculated that chocolate—America's favorite addiction—similarly releases serotonin as well as endorphins, the brain's natural painkillers.[2] It's little wonder, then, that when we feel stressed, we medicate ourselves with big bowls of pasta or chocolate bars or mounds of mashed potatoes—all thought of, appropriately enough, as "comfort foods." (Not that I want to malign dark chocolate—in small doses, it has some wonderful ingredients that reduce inflammation and are good for your heart.) The benefits of dark chocolate notwithstanding, what you eat does very much impact your moods. What you don't eat is also a factor!

A friend of mine says, "A hungry man is an angry man." Hunger makes people grouchy—no question. We call it "hangry." Low blood sugar is the culprit. When those levels drop, people find it difficult to concentrate. For some, low blood sugar evolves into what feels like a life-threatening situation, especially if glucose levels go down far enough. These individuals can experience lightheadedness, confusion, heart palpitations, sweating, lack of energy, and other alarming symptoms. It's easy to see how such a person would become aggressive, especially where food is concerned.[3] But even if your physiology doesn't unravel to that degree—hunger can make you grumpy and interfere with your finding Moodtopia.

Many women become moody simply because they're deficient in protein. That's why I recommend to my clients that they consume protein three times a day. This helps them feel satiated and it ensures that their blood sugar levels remain stable. The following recipes include high-protein snacks and "power balls" and some that contain herbs. These will give you the quick pick-me-up you need when you feel yourself sinking into an episode of "hangriness"—especially if you're too busy to stop and eat a decent meal.

It's equally important to stay hydrated. Two recent studies at the University of Connecticut's Human Performance Laboratory found that the participants' mental, mood, and cognitive capacities were impacted by even mild dehydration (which they defined as only a 1.5% loss in the body's normal water volume). And it didn't even matter whether their healthy, active young subjects had walked on a treadmill for forty minutes or were sitting still. The negative effects of mild dehydration were identical.[4]

Alleviating hunger or thirst is vitally important to maintaining Moodtopia, as these states can remain invisible to you. Only after having eaten or sipped some water, may you realize that nutrition (or lack thereof) was dampening your mood. However, over the years, I've found that the food-mood connection can be further refined. The following recipes include some of my favorite drinks and quick snacks that will help you in your quest to be less moody. Although it is always best to sit down for a balanced meal in a calm environment where you are relaxed and chewing your food properly, this may not always be possible. That's when a quick sip of a healthy drink and downing a super protein-packed nut snack, or quickly dunking a rice cake into a nutritious dip can make all the difference.

BLACKSTRAP MOLASSES POWER DRINK

What is blackstrap molasses? It's created when sugarcane is boiled down three times. It is lower in sugar than other types of molasses, because each boiling of the cane removes more sugar. Herbalists consider blackstrap molasses to be the poor man's multivitamin. (But all people rich or poor can benefit from it!) It's inexpensive and easy to use.

You may be wondering why I am suggesting you use an ingredient that has sugar. Well, blackstrap molasses is one of the few sweeteners containing vitamins and minerals. It's very high in iron (which provides energy and boosts metabolism) without being constipating and it's rich in calcium. It also contains such minerals as copper, potassium, zinc, selenium, manganese, and the very important magnesium as well as vitamin B_6, niacin, and pantothenic acid. I consider blackstrap molasses a superfood and a great tool in your quest for Moodtopia. I like my clients to have a cup of warm Blackstrap Molasses Power Drink every morning because I know they'll begin their day with tons of minerals often missing in our modern diet. This quick and nutritious morning drink can chase the tiredness out of your body and give you a boost. My favorite recipe is simple and takes only a few minutes to prepare. In the summer you can also drink this iced.

SERVING: 1

1 tablespoon blackstrap molasses
1 tablespoon honey
1 cup hot water
A splash of rice, almond, or hemp milk

Combine the ingredients and serve hot or chilled.

SARA-CHANA'S FAMOUS PUNCH

I love to have this tea in the fridge at all times because dehydration can contribute to moodiness. The magic ingredients are blueberry or black cherry concentrates that are so rich in antioxidants, especially flavonoids. In a study of nearly 300,000 Canadians, greater fruit and vegetable consumption was associated with lower odds of depression, psychological distress, self-reported mood and anxiety disorders, and poor perceived mental health. The researchers conclude that since a healthy diet comprised of a high intake of fruits and vegetables is rich in antioxidants, it may consequently dampen the detrimental effects of oxidative stress on mental health.[5] Besides, this is my kids' favorite drink, and all the other children in our building love it, too. It tastes like punch but is healthy, nutritious, and hydrating. It's delicious and refreshing, too!

MAKES 64 OUNCES; 20 TO 30 SERVINGS

> 6 to 8 tea bags (I usually use Celestial Seasonings Black Cherry
> Zinger or Red Raspberry Zinger, but any flavor will work)
>
> 2 cups boiled, filtered water
>
> 2 to 4 tablespoons honey (to taste)
>
> ½ cup black cherry or blueberry concentrate (I use Dynamic
> Health brand)
>
> 1½ quarts cold filtered water (replace some of the water with ice
> cubes, if desired)

1. Place the tea bags in a 64-ounce heatproof pitcher and cover them with the boiled, filtered water.
2. Allow to steep for 20 minutes.
3. Stir well, then add honey to taste, the fruit concentrate, filtered water, and ice, if desired.
4. Refrigerate *and enjoy.*

ROSEMARY GLADSTAR'S ENERGY HERB ZOOM BALLS

This alternative to caffeine drinks was developed by herbalist Rosemary Gladstar, author of *Herbs for Stress & Anxiety*. Rosemary says that "These energy balls are full of nourishing herbs that support overall well-being. And with the addition of guarana and kola, they give us that extra zoom to help lift our spirits and get us through the day. However, it is important to recognize that both guarana and kola nut are caffeine-rich and are not recommended for people who suffered from long-term undiagnosed exhaustion. Using them occasionally for energy is fine. One to two balls will 'brighten your brain.'" Guarana powder is high in caffeine but has only one alkaloid compared with the thirteen in coffee.

SERVINGS: 20 TO 25

3 ounces guarana powder (see note)

1 ounce kola nut powder (see note)

1 ounce bee pollen (see note)

2 ounces Siberian ginseng (see note)

¼ teaspoon ground nutmeg, coriander, or cardamom (optional, for flavor—choose one)

1 cup tahini or sesame butter (or other nut butter)

½ cup honey

1 cup chocolate or carob chips (or more, to taste)

6 ounces unsweetened shredded coconut

¼ cup chopped walnuts or almonds

Unsweetened carob powder

1. In a medium-size bowl, stir the herbs and bee pollen into the tahini and stir in the honey.
2. Add the chocolate chips, coconut, and nuts.
3. Thicken the mixture with the unsweetened carob powder.

4. Scoop small spoonfuls and squeeze each tightly in the palm of your hand, then roll into small balls.

5. Place in a plastic container that can be sealed tightly, and store in a cool place.

NOTE: Although we don't discuss these herbs, they're recommended by herbalists worldwide to boost energy and stamina. They are best bought in powdered form from Mountain Rose Herbs or Frontier Co-op.

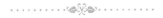

ENERGY HERB ZOOM BALLS #2

SERVINGS: 20 TO 25

½ cup any type nut butter, such as almond, cashew, sunflower seed, or peanut

½ cup honey

¼ cup astragalus powder (see note)

¼ cup eleuthero powder

¼ cup ashwagandha powder

1 tablespoon licorice powder (see note)

1 tablespoon ground ginger (see note)

1 tablespoon ground cardamom or fennel (see note)

1. In a large bowl, mix together the nut butter of your choice and the honey.

2. In a second bowl, stir together all the powdered and ground herbs.

3. Reserving a small amount of the herb mixture for dusting, slowly mix the herb mixture into the nut butter mixture until a thick paste forms.

4. Roll into balls 1 inch in diameter.

5. Dust with the reserved herb mixture to prevent sticking.

6. Store in the refrigerator in airtight container.

NOTE: Although we don't discuss these herbs, they're recommended by herbalists worldwide to boost energy and stamina.

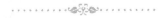

NUT PROTEIN BALLS

Nuts are high in protein and are a great emotional pick-me-up! They're also an excellent source of vitamin E, magnesium, phosphorus, copper, manganese, and selenium. In addition, many nuts are high in tryptophan, an essential amino acid that has been found useful in reducing general anxiety, social anxiety disorder, and panic attacks. Tryptophan is needed to synthesize serotonin, a neurotransmitter dubbed the "happy molecule." Serotonin plays a large role in mood, sleep, learning, and appetite control. Low serotonin levels are widely believed to be a major cause of depression.

Most of my clients are constantly on the run. Protein bars are all the rage, and it's helpful to eat them between proper meals, especially to avoid "hangriness." I teach my clients to make these and the following protein balls. They're easy, convenient, healthier than store-bought, and are mood boosters, too! You might want to add some ground cinnamon (for flavor and its blood sugar–regulating properties) or ground ginger (for its help with digestion). You can also add turmeric, which is a great antioxidant, but just be aware that it can stain fingers (and possibly clothes) bright yellow.

SERVINGS: 20

2 cups walnuts or any other nut or seed

1 cup shredded unsweetened coconut, plus more for rolling (optional)

2 cups soft pitted dates (Medjool are the yummiest)

2 tablespoons light olive oil

1 teaspoon sea salt

1 teaspoon pure vanilla extract

½ cup shredded coconut or cocoa powder (optional)

1. Process the walnuts and coconut in a large food processor fitted with an S-blade until crumbly. Add the dates, oil, sea salt, and vanilla and process again until a sticky batter is formed.
2. Scoop the dough by heaping tablespoons and roll between your hands to form balls. You can leave the balls the way they are or roll them in either shredded coconut or cocoa powder.
3. Store the balls in a sealed container in the refrigerator for up to 2 to 3 weeks. Or you can freeze them for 3 months.

NUT CHIA BALLS #1

Chia seeds are a great food to stabilize moods. The word *chia* means "strength" in ancient Mayan. Warriors used the seeds to boost their energy and increase stamina. Just a tablespoon is helpful because these seeds have a lot of fiber, omega-3 fatty acids, calcium, high-quality plant-based protein, minerals, and antioxidants. Omega-3 fatty acids and calcium are essential nutrients for the life of a neuron and ease anxiety, depression, and irritability. The electrical pulses within the nervous system depend on calcium to perform properly. When a calcium deficiency compromises the nervous system, chances of irregular moods and anxiety attacks increase significantly. Chia seeds also absorb liquid, forming a gel that helps coat the stomach and intestines, aiding digestion.

SERVINGS: 20 TO 25

1 cup almond flour

¼ cup sesame seeds

¼ cup chia seeds

¼ cup raw cacao or unsweetened cocoa powder

½ cup any type nut butter, such as almond, cashew, sunflower seed, or peanut

1 tablespoon light olive oil

2 to 3 tablespoons pure maple syrup

½ teaspoon ground cinnamon or ginger (optional)

Optional coating: sesame seeds, cacao nibs, coconut flakes, sunflower seeds, or chia seeds

1. Combine all the ingredients, except the optional coating, in a food processor and process until well blended. The consistency should be crumbly and pastelike.

2. Scoop small spoonfuls and squeeze each tightly in the palm of your hand, then roll into small balls.

3. Serve plain or roll in sesame seeds, cacao nibs, coconut flakes, sunflower seeds, or chia seeds.

4. Store in an airtight container in the fridge for up to a week. Refrigerating them will make them firmer.

NUT CHIA BALLS #2

Oats are among the most nutrient-dense foods you can eat. They are rich in protein, good fats, and fiber. They are filled with vitamins and minerals—especially B vitamins—which keep the brain and nervous system healthy and help maintain energy levels. Oats are calming and invigorating at the same time. That's one of the reasons they're fed to racehorses. Horses need to be calm and centered, but need energy to race. And that is exactly what we want for ourselves!

SERVINGS: 20 TO 25

1 cup rolled oats

1 cup unsweetened coconut flakes

½ cup chia seeds (see note)

½ cup dark chocolate chips

½ cup any type nut butter, such as almond, cashew, sunflower seed, or peanut

⅓ cup honey

1 teaspoon pure vanilla extract, rum extract, or orange extract

½ teaspoon ground cinnamon or ginger (optional)

1. Place all the ingredients in a bowl or food processer and mix well.
2. Refrigerate for about 90 minutes.
3. Scoop small spoonfuls and squeeze each tightly in the palm of your hand, then roll into small balls.
4. Store in an airtight container in the fridge for up to a week.

NOTE: *If you are concerned about chia seeds getting stuck in your teeth, feel free to use ground chia or grind them in a coffee grinder or small food processor.*

ALMOND DATE ENERGY BALLS

SERVINGS: 20 TO 25

2 cups raw almonds

2 cups pitted dates, preferably Medjool

¼ cup honey

Light olive oil, for forming balls

1. Grind the almonds in a food processor until finely chopped, then transfer to a baking pan.
2. Add the pitted dates to the food processor and pulse until finely chopped and the mixture forms a ball. Transfer from the processor to a bowl.
3. Add half of the ground almonds to the dates, reserving the remaining ground almonds on the baking pan.
4. Add honey to the date mixture and mix until smooth.
5. Coat your hands with a little oil so it's easy to form the mixture into balls, then roll each in the reserved chopped almonds to coat well.
6. Place the balls in a tightly sealed container until ready to eat.
7. Any leftover chopped nuts can be sprinkled over the balls to keep them from sticking if transporting.
8. Will keep for up to 5 days at room temperature or up to a week, if refrigerated.

CREAMY GARLIC TOFU DIP

It is so important to eat lots of vegetables, because they keep moods in check. But many of my clients complain that they just don't like them. I encourage them to make delicious dips. I find that helps them eat the vegetables they need.

Tofu is a great way to obtain protein when you are on the run. It's also an excellent source of iron and has high amounts of calcium, vitamin E, and phytonutrients. Tofu also has zero cholesterol and few carbs. This dip is full of phytoestrogens and will help balance a woman in a tasty way. It's delicious served with rye, spelt, or rice crackers or raw veggies. This is easy to snack on at work or between meals as a pick-me-up.

SERVINGS: 6

2 tablespoons sunflower seeds

2 garlic cloves

10 baby spinach leaves

1 (14-ounce) tub soft or silken tofu

2 teaspoons toasted sesame oil

1 tablespoon rice vinegar

½ teaspoon dry mustard

½ teaspoon sea salt

1. Place the sunflower seeds, garlic, and spinach in a blender and pulse for a few seconds.
2. Add the remaining ingredients and mix on low speed for 1 minute.
3. Eat immediately with raw vegetables or refrigerate and store for later use. Will keep for 1 week in the fridge.

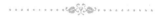

SUNFLOWER SEED HERBAL DIP

Sunflower seeds are an excellent source of protein, amino acids, calcium, magnesium, and tryptophan. They are also one of the best sources of B vitamins, including niacin, folic acid, thiamine (vitamin B_1), pyridoxine (vitamin B_6), pantothenic acid, and riboflavin. All the B vitamins are beneficial for the brain. Vitamin B_6 is especially important for regulating moods and preventing mental fatigue. B vitamins are also needed for the brain to produce the important feel-good neurotransmitter serotonin that lifts your spirits. The seeds' high level of magnesium balances calcium, helping to regulate nerve function, and the amino acid tryptophan also enhances serotonin production.

MAKES ABOUT 3 CUPS

2 cups organic, hulled sunflower seeds, raw or roasted

2 garlic cloves

2 teaspoons cider vinegar or rice vinegar

Juice of ½ lemon

1 tablespoon chopped fresh parsley, or 1 teaspoon dried

1 tablespoon chopped fresh dill, or 1 teaspoon dried

1 tablespoon dried thyme

1½ teaspoons dried sage

1 tablespoon chopped fresh basil, or 1 tsp dried

1 cup organic mayonnaise

1. In a food processor, process the sunflower seeds until they obtain the consistency of chunky peanut butter. Transfer to a bowl.

2. Add the garlic, vinegar, lemon juice, herbs, and mayo and mix gently by hand.

3. Serve as a dip with raw vegetables.

ACKNOWLEDGMENTS

THIS BOOK WOULD HAVE BEEN IMPOSSIBLE WITHOUT THE SUPPORT, ASSISTANCE, AND ENCOURagement of the special people in my life.

I'd like to begin by thanking Jerry Bluestein and Regine Wood for being the first to encourage me to turn my fantasies of writing a book, appearing on TV shows, and becoming a keynote speaker into reality. They told me that I needed to stop dreaming and go out there and make it happen! They were the ones who introduced me to one of my favorite writers, Susan Golant. I had read all of Susan's parenting books and was an all-time groupie. And then, as luck and fate would have it, she became my writing partner. What an honor!

I am grateful to my daughter Bruryah, who, through all the chaos in our lives, has always been able to help me keep my life, schedule, and office up and running, all while watching over her younger siblings like a lioness. Sima Leah Duato and Chana Goldreich were my backstage hands who were there for me all the time, day and night, and in between. I am forever grateful to my dear and wonderful friends Shaya and Chanie Gordon, my biggest cheerleaders, who helped me hire James Weir from the Anderson Group, the incredible publicist who got this project rolling. Life coach Dr. Joel Kreisberg helped give me the strength to be proud of my successes and use my bursting energy constructively. Dr. Kreisberg also assisted with the production of my app, "Sara-Chana's Savvy Breastfeeding Guide."

A big thank-you to Mayer Bendet, who was patient with my babbling and was there for me all the time. My sincerest appreciation to Yittie and Dovid Tabak, who helped me actualize my vision, and Etti and Moshe Drizin, who believed in me. I'm also grateful

Acknowledgments

to Bracha Meshchaninov, who hosted me as I put the last touches on *Moodtopia*, Yehudis Chana Meshchaninov, who kept my mind together during this hectic time, and Maria, who kept my home together.

My two magical managers—truly my gift—Milt Suchin and Dann Moss of the Carpe Diem Group LLC—introduced me to my fabulous and insightful book agent, Dan Strone from Trident Media Group; he saw the potential in my book and presented it to a most impressive and esteemed editor, Renée Sedliar, at Da Capo Press. Renée is smart, savvy, and every correction and insight was right on the mark; I have the greatest respect for her and her enchanted touch. I'm also grateful to Rivka Freeman who designed my Cycle of Sanity charts.

But the real heroes of this project are my husband, Avrohom, who gave me the space to pursue my dreams and is forever patient with my ambitions and goals. My sisters, Hilary and Shayne, give me their unconditional love, which is more important than anything. And I would not have been encouraged to research and write about moods without my amazing, gifted, generous children: Bruryah, Moshe Chayim, Menachem Nochum, Shneur Zalman, Shmuel Dovid, Shimshon Leib, and Shifrah. They educated me in ways no university ever could. I love them so deeply with every cell of my body. I thank my kids for being tolerant of their overzealous and persistently passionate mother.

—Sara-Chana Silverstein, RH (AHG), IBCLC
Brooklyn, New York. February 2018

FOR MY PART, I, TOO, AM MOST GRATEFUL TO JERRY BLUESTEIN AND REGINE WOOD FOR introducing me to the force of nature known as Sara-Chana Silverstein, a bright, energetic woman with a unique voice and perspective. Working with Sara-Chana has been enlightening and entertaining—she has added richly to my life. I'm also grateful to our editor, Renée Sedliar, for her meticulous attention to our manuscript, enthusiastic support, incisive comments, and astute guidance. She has made this process most enjoyable. As always, I thank my agents Richard Pine and Eliza Rothstein at Inkwell Management for carefully overseeing my interests. And I am forever grateful to my husband, Dr. Mitch Golant, without whom none of this would be possible.

—Susan K. Golant, MA
Los Angeles, California. February 2018

RESOURCES

HERB PURVEYORS

Eclectic Herbs https://www.eclecticherb.com/

Frontier Co-op https://www.frontiercoop.com/bulk-herbs-and-teas/herbs/

Gaia Herbs http://GaiaHerbs.com/

Hawaii Pharm https://www.hawaiipharm.com/index.php?route=common/home/

Healing Spirit Farm http://healingspiritsherbfarm.com/

Herb Pharm http://www.herb-pharm.com/

Herbalist and Alchemist http://www.herbalist-alchemist.com/

Herbs Etc. http://www.herbsetc.com/

Herbs of Light https://www.herbsoflight.com/

Herb Lore https://herblore.com/

Mountain Rose Herbs https://www.mountainroseherbs.com/

Planetary Herbals http://www.planetaryherbals.com/

Standard Process https://www.standardprocess.com/

Urban Moonshine https://www.urbanmoonshine.com/

WishGarden Herbs http://www.wishgardenherbs.com/

Woodland Essence https://woodlandessence.com/

ESSENTIAL OIL PURVEYORS

Art Naturals https://artnaturals.com/

Aura Cacia https://www.auracacia.com/

Doterra https://www.doterra.com/US/en/

Mountain Rose Herbs https://www.mountainroseherbs.com/

New Directions Aromatics https://www.newdirectionsaromatics.com/

Plant Therapy https://www.planttherapy.com/

Snow Lotus http://www.snowlotus.org/

Young Living https://www.living-essential-oils.com/

NOTES

CHAPTER 2: UNDERSTANDING THE "CYCLE-OF-SANITY"

1. Personal communication, April 2017.

2. Mitch Golant and Susan Golant, *What to Do When Someone You Love Is Depressed: A Practical, Compassionate, and Helpful Guide* (New York: Holt, 2007): 22–26.

3. Alex Lickerman, "The Benefit of Sadness," *Psychology Today*, March 4, 2012, https://www.psychologytoday.com/us/blog/happiness-in-world/201203/the-benefit-sadness.

4. Kathleen Doheny, "Why We Cry: The Truth About Tearing Up," WebMD, October 30, 2000, https://www.webmd.com/balance/features/why-we-cry-the-truth-about-tearing-up#1.

5. Golant and Golant, *What to Do When Someone You Love Is Depressed*.

6. Personal communication, January 2018.

7. Marie A, "Four Sacred Plants," Redroad Collective Newsletter, June 17, 2009, http://www.oocities.org/redroadcollective/SacredTobacco.html.

8. Candace Pert, *Molecules of Emotion: The Science Behind Mind-Body Medicine* (New York: Touchstone: 1999), cited in "Where Do You Store Your Emotions?" www.candacepert.com/where-do-you-store-your-emotions.

9. Personal communication, June 8, 2016.

10. Srikumar Rao, *Happiness at Work: Be Resilient, Motivated, and Successful—No Matter What* (New York: McGraw-Hill, 2010).

CHAPTER 3: CHARTING YOUR MOODS

1. Personal communication, April 2016.

CHAPTER 4: NOURISH YOUR LIVER AND REVITALIZE WITH ADAPTOGENS

1. Avi Solomon, "The Regimen of Health by Moses Maimonides," Medium Learning for Life, 2014, https://medium.com/learning-for-life/the-regimen-of-health-by-moses-maimonides-d5c22244fc5a.

2. Personal communication, December 2016.

3. M. Ananya Mandal, "Adrenal Gland Function," News-Medical.net, 2011, https://www.news-medical.net/health/What-Does-the-Adrenal-Gland-Do.aspx.

4. Marty Nemko, PhD, "From Stress to Genes, Baboons to Hormones," *Psychology Today*, February 4, 2017, https://www.psychologytoday.com/us/blog/how-do-life/201702/stress-genes-baboons-hormones.

5. Bill Hathaway, "Yale Team Discovers How Stress and Depression Can Shrink the Brain," *YaleNews*, August 12, 2012, https://news.yale.edu/2012/08/12/yale-team-discovers-how-stress-and-depression-can-shrink-brain.

6. Martha Nolte Kennedy, "The Liver & Blood Sugar," Collective Work 2007–2018, https://dtc.ucsf.edu/types-of-diabetes/type2/understanding-type-2-diabetes/how-the-body-processes-sugar/the-liver-blood-sugar/.

7. University of Gothenburg, "Permanent Stress Can Cause Type 2 Diabetes in Men, Study Suggests," ScienceDaily, February 7, 2013, https://www.sciencedaily.com/releases/2013/02/130207114418.htm.

8. Alan Franciscus, "Stress and the Liver," HCV Advocate, accessed July 2017, http://hcvadvocate.org/hepatitis/factsheetsB_pdf/stress_liver.pdf.

9. Personal communication, May 2017.

10. Susun S. Weed, "Nourishing the Liver the Wise Woman Way," 2018, http://www.exploringwomanhood.com/mindbodysoul/health/liver-health.htm.

11. E-mail interview, February 24, 2016.

12. Personal communication, February 21, 2016.

13. Personal communication, February 9, 2016.

14. Guido Masé, *The Wild Medicine Solution: Healing with Aromatic, Bitter, and Tonic Plants* (Randolph, VT: Healing Arts Press, 2013).

15. Personal communication, February 7, 2016.

16. Personal communication from Guido Masé, February 10, 2016.

17. Steven D. Ehrlich, "Anemia," University of New Mexico, December 19, 2015, http://www.umm.edu/health/medical/altmed/condition/anemia.

18. David Winston, "Harmony Remedies: An Overview of Adaptogens," Herbalstudies.net, accessed August 2017, https://www.herbalstudies.net/_media/resources/library/HarmonyRemedies(1).pdf.

19. Personal communication, November 16, 2017.

20. Kristina Johnson, "Before Steroids, Russians Secretly Studied Herbs," August 19, 2016, https://www.nationalgeographic.com/people-and-culture/food/the-plate/2016/08/long-before-doping-scandals-russians-were-studying-performance-/.

21. David Winston, *Adaptogens: Herbs for Strength, Stamina, and Stress Relief* (Randolph, VT: Healing Arts Press, 2007).

CHAPTER 5: MOOD HERBS TO THE RESCUE

1. "Herbs at a Glance," NCCIH, 2011, https://nccih.nih.gov/health/herbsataglance.htm.

2. Ibid.

3. Donnie Yance, MH, CN, "Kava: Natural Relief for Anxiety," January 31, 2014, http://www.donnieyance.com/kava-natural-relief-anxiety/.

4. Personal communication, May 25, 2016.

5. "Children's Dosage Guide," Herb Lore, accessed July 2017, https://herblore.com/overviews/childrens-dosage-guide.

6. Personal communication, May 2017.

7. Personal communication, July 2017.

8. Steven D. Ehrlich, "St. John's Wort," University of Maryland Medical Center, accessed June 2017, http://www.umm.edu/health/medical/altmed/herb/st-johns-wort; Jennifer Grebow, "A Warning Label for St. John's Wort?" *Nutritional Outlook*, February 8, 2012, http://www.nutritionaloutlook.com/herbs-botanicals/warning-label-st-johns-wort.

9. Office of Dietary Supplements, "Valerian," accessed June 2017, National Institutes of Health, https://ods.od.nih.gov/factsheets/Valerian-HealthProfessional/.

CHAPTER 6: AROMATHERAPY: SCENTS-ING YOUR WAY TO SERENITY

1. Robert Tisserand, "Gattefossé's Burn," April 22, 2011, http://roberttisserand.com/2011/04/gattefosses-burn/.

2. Kang-Ming Chang and Chuh-Wei Shen, "Aromatherapy Benefits Autonomic Nervous System Regulation for Elementary School Faculty in Taiwan," *Evidence-Based Complementary and Alternative Medicine* (2011): 1–7, doi:10.1155/2011/946537, https://www.hindawi.com/journals/ecam/2011/946537/.

3. Rachel S. Herz, "Do Scents Affect People's Moods or Work Performance?" *Scientific American* (November 2002), accessed 2018, https://www.scientificamerican.com/article/do-scents-affect-peoples-/.

4. Ibid.

5. Cynthia Deng, "Aromatherapy: Exploring Olfaction," *Yale Scientific Magazine*, November 16, 2011, http://www.yalescientific.org/2011/11/aromatherapy-exploring-olfaction/.

6. Ibid.

7. Betty Vine, "Aromatherapy and the Brain: Part 2. Brain World," *Brain World*, June 29, 2015, http://brainworldmagazine.com/aromatherapy-and-the-brain-part-2/.

8. The UC Berkeley lab scientist Noam Sobel found when examining the influence of smelling coffee on olfactory habituation, "Smelling coffee aroma between perfume samples, as compared to smelling unscented air, actually works. The perceived odor intensity of the perfume from sample to sample stayed the same after smelling coffee aroma while it decreased when smelling air between samples. The pleasantness of the perfume, however, was similar after smelling coffee or air." BeanPoster, "Coffee 'Nose' Best! Does Coffee Cleanse Our Nasal Palate?" January 2, 2013, https://www.theroasterie.com/blog/coffee-nose-best-does-coffee-cleanse-our-nasal-palate/.

9. Personal communication, October 2017.

CHAPTER 7: FAKING IT

1. Personal communication, November 16, 2017.

2. Random Acts of Kindness Foundation. "Benefits of RAK," http://mailstat.us/tr/t/y8a2fvvqjd14zqq9/1e/https://www.randomactsofkindness.org/the-science-of-kindness.

3. Christine Carter, *Raising Happiness: 10 Simple Steps for More Joyful Kids and Happier Parents* (New York: Ballantine Books, 2010).

4. Stephen Post, "The Science of Kindness: How Practicing Kindness Benefits Overall Well-Being," Health & Wellness Magazine, Mid-Tennessee Edition, accessed February 5, 2018, http://tnhealthandwellness.com/the-science-of-kindness-how-practicing-kindness-benefits-overall-well-being/.

5. Carter, *Raising Happiness*.

6. Irene Conlan, "How You Benefit When You Pay It Forward with Random Acts of Kindness," January 30, 2018, https://theselfimprovementblog.com/self-improvement/love-and-relationships/do-you-remember-pay-it-forward/.

7. Jill Ladwig, "Brain Can Be Trained in Compassion, Study Shows," May 22, 2013, http://news.wisc.edu/brain-can-be-trained-in-compassion-study-shows/#sthash.ipNcuhAs.dpuf.

8. Christian Jarrett, "Smiling Changes How You View the World," *New York Magazine*, April 6, 2015.

9. James D. Laird, *Feelings: The Perception of Self* (New York: Oxford University Press: 2007).

10. James D. Laird, "Self-attribution of Emotion: The Effects of Expressive Behavior on the Quality of Emotional Experience," *Journal of Personality and Social Psychology* (May 1974), doi:10.1037/h0036125.

11. Sarah Stevenson, "There's Magic in Your Smile: How Smiling Affects Your Brain," *Psychology Today*, June 25, 2012.

12. Ibid.

13. Jarrett, "Smiling Changes How You View the World."

14. Ibid.

15. Alejandra Sel, Beatriz Calvo-Merino, Simone Tuettenberg, and Bettinga Forster, "When You Smile, the World Smiles at You: ERP Evidence for Self-expression Effects on Face Processing," *Social Cognitive and Affective Neuroscience* 10, no. 10: 1316–1322, doi:10.1093/scan/nsv009.

16. Daily Mail Reporter, "Average Adult Manages Seven Smiles a Day…But One Is False!" March 3, 2013, updated March 5, 2013, http://www.dailymail.co.uk/news/article-2288833/Average-adult-manages-seven-smiles-day-false.html.

17. William Fry. "Laugh Yourself Healthy," June 7, 2014, https://laughyourselfhealthy.wordpress.com/tag/dr-william-fry/.

18. Adrienne Weeks, "How Many Calories Do You Burn Each Time You Laugh?" July 18, 2017, https://www.livestrong.com/article/308619-how-many-calories-do-you-burn-each-time-you-laugh/.

19. "Laughter Is the Best Medicine," HelpGuide.org, accessed February 5, 2018, https://www.helpguide.org/articles/mental-health/laughter-is-the-best-medicine.htm.

20. Schloma Majeski, *The Chassidic Approach to Joy* (self-published, 1995).

21. Mitch Golant and Susan Golant, *What to Do When Someone You Love is Depressed: A Practical, Compassionate, and Helpful Guide* (New York: Holt, 2007), 117.

22. Viktor E. Frankl, *Man's Search for Meaning* (Boston: Beacon Press, 2006).

CHAPTER 8: USING YOUR INTUITIVE SELF TO REACH MOODTOPIA

1. Luanne Brizendine, *The Female Brain* (New York: Morgan Road Books, 2006).

2. Judith Orloff, *Dr. Judith Orloff's Guide to Intuitive Healing: Five Steps to Physical, Emotional, and Sexual Wellness* (New York: Crown, 2000).

3. Gerard P. Hodgkinson, Janice Langan-Fox, and Eugene Sadler-Smith, "Intuition: A Fundamental Bridging Construct in the Behavioural Sciences," *British Journal of Psychology* 99 (2008): 1–27, http://onlinelibrary.wiley.com/doi/10.1348/000712607X216666/epdf?r3_referer=wol&tracking_action=preview_click&show_checkout=1&purchase_referrer=search.yahoo.

4. Jennifer Wolkin, "Meet Your Second Brain: The Gut," *Mindful*, August 14, 2015, https://www.mindful.org/meet-your-second-brain-the-gut;   https://www.psychologytoday.com/articles/201111/your-backup-brain; Dan Hurley, "Your Backup Brain," *Psychology Today*, November 1, 2011, https://www.psychologytoday.com/articles/201111/your-backup-brain.

5. Colleen Oakley, "The Power of Female Intuition," WebMD, 2012, http://www.webmd.com/balance/features/power-of-female-intuition#1.

6. Adam Hadhazy, "Think Twice: How the Gut's 'Second Brain' Influences Mood and Well-Being," *Scientific American*, February 12, 2010, https://www.scientificamerican.com/article/gut-second-brain/.

7. Emeran Mayer, *The Mind-Gut Connection: How the Hidden Conversation Within Our Bodies Impacts Our Mood, Our Choices, and Our Overall Health* (New York: Harper Wave, 2016).

8. Brizendine *The Female Brain*.

9. Luanne Brizendine, "The Female Brain," *New York Times*, September 10, 2016, http://www.nytimes.com/2006/09/10/books/chapters/0910-1st-briz.html.

10. Sherrie Dillard, "Three Ways to Make the Most of Women's Intuition," http://omtimes.com/2012/08/three-ways-to-make-the-most-of-womens-intuition/.

11. The Personal Safety Training Group, "What Is Situational Awareness?" http://www.personalsafetygroup.com/about/situational-awareness-training/.

12. Audrey Nelson and Susan K. Golant, *You Don't Say: Navigating Nonverbal Communication Between the Sexes* (New York: Berkley Publishing Group, 2004), 2–3.

13. Alice Mado Proverbio, Marta Calbi, Mirella Manfredi, and Alberto Zani, "Comprehending Body Language and Mimics: An ERP and Neuroimaging Study on Italian Actors and Viewers," PLoS One 9, no. 3 (2014): e91294.

14. Elizabeth Norton Lasley, "The Hormone That Calms and Connects. The Oxytocin Factor: Tapping the Hormone of Calm, Love, and Healing," Dana Foundation, January 1, 2004, http://www.dana.org/Cerebrum/2004/The_Hormone_That_Calms_and_Connects/.

15. "Study: Choosing a Home Close to Nature Improves Mental Health for Years," Wilderness Society, January 29, 2014, http://wilderness.org/blog/study-choosing-home-close-nature-improves-mental-health-years; Daniel T. C. Cox, Danielle F. Shanahan, Hannah L. Hudson, Kate E. Plummer, Gavin M. Siriwardena, Richard A. Fuller, Karen Anderson, Steven Hancock, and Kevin J. Gaston, "Doses of Neighborhood Nature: The Benefits for Mental Health of Living with Nature," *BioScience* 67, no. 2 (February 1, 2017): 147–155, https://doi.org/10.1093/biosci/biw173, https://academic.oup.com/bioscience/article/67/2/147/2900179/Doses-of-Neighborhood-Nature-The-Benefits-for.

16. Jean Larson and Mary Jo Kreitzer, "How Does Nature Impact Our Wellbeing?" University of Minnesota, https://www.takingcharge.csh.umn.edu/enhance-your-well-being/environment/nature-and-us/how-does-nature-impact-our-well-being.

17. Ruth Ann Atchley, David L. Strayer, and Paul Atchley. "Creativity in the Wild: Improving Creative Reasoning Through Immersion in Natural Settings," *PloS One* 7, no. 12 (December 12, 2012): e51474, https://doi.org/10.1371/journal.pone.0051474.

18. Deborah Franklin, "How Hospital Gardens Help Patients Heal," *Scientific American*, March 1, 2012, accessed 2018, https://www.scientificamerican.com/article/nature-that-nurtures/.

CHAPTER 9: FINDING AND CREATING SPACES THAT HELP YOU FEEL GOOD

1. Personal communication, July 14, 2017.

2. Marie Kondo, *The Life-Changing Magic of Tidying Up: The Japanese Art of Decluttering and Organizing* (San Francisco: Ten Speed Press, 2014).

3. Steven Masley, *The 30-Day Heart Tune-Up* (New York: Center Street, 2014), 179.

4. Richard Louv, *Last Child in the Woods: Saving Our Children from Nature-Deficit Disorder* (New York: Algonquin Books, 2008).

5. Marlys Harris, "Kids Stay Indoors: What Happened to, 'Go Outside and Play'?" Minn-Post, August 8, 2013, accessed 2018, https://www.minnpost.com/cityscape/2013/08/kids-stay-indoors-what-happened-go-outside-and-play.

6. Florian Lederbogen, Peter Kirsch, Leila Haddad, Fabian Streit, Heike Tost, Philipp Schuch, Stefan Wüst, Jens C. Pruessner, Marcella Rietschel, Michael Deuschle, and Andreas Meyer-Lindenberg "City Living and Urban Upbringing Affect Neural Social Stress Processing in Humans," Nature 474, no. 7352 (June 22, 2011): 498–501, doi:10.1038/nature 10190.http://www.nature.com/nature/journal/v474/n7352/full/nature10190.html?foxtrotcallback=true.

7. Ibid.

8. Gretchen Reynolds, "How Walking In Nature Changes the Brain," New York Times (blog), July 22, 2015, https://well.blogs.nytimes.com/2015/07/22/how-nature-changes-the-brain/.

9. Florence Williams, "This Is Your Brain on Nature," National Geographic, January 2016, http://www.nationalgeographic.com/magazine/2016/01/call-to-wild/.

10. Ibid.

11. Florence Williams, "Benefits of Nature: How Nature Helps Your Brain," Reader's Digest, April 2017, http://www.rd.com/health/wellness/benefits-of-nature/.

12. Yuko Tsunetsugu, Bum-Jin Park, and Yoshifumi Miyazaki, "Trends in Research Related to 'Shinrin-Yoku' (Taking in the Forest Atmosphere or Forest Bathing) in Japan," Environmental Health and Preventive Medicine 15 (January 15, 2010): 27–37, doi:10.1007/s12199-009-0091-z, https://www.ncbi.nlm.nih.gov/pmc/articles/PMC2793347/; http://www.shinrin-yoku.org/shinrin-yoku.html; Meeri Kim, "'Forest Bathing' Is Latest Fitness Trend to Hit U.S.—

'Where Yoga Was 30 Years Ago,'" *Washington Post*, May 17, 2016, accessed 2018, https://www
.washingtonpost.com/news/to-your-health/wp/2016/05/17/forest-bathing-is-latest
-fitness-trend-to-hit-u-s-where-yoga-was-30-years-ago/?utm_term=.b1e9e6f734be.

13. "Forest Bathing," HpHp Central, accessed April 2017, http://www.hphpcentral.com
/article/forest-bathing; https://hikingresearch.wordpress.com/tag/dr-qing-li/.

14. Catharine Paddock, "Soil Bacteria Work in Similar Way to Antidepressants," *Medical
News Today*, April 2, 2007, http://www.medicalnewstoday.com/articles/66840.php; Bonnie L.
Grant, "Antidepressant Microbes in Soil: How Dirt Makes You Happy," August 25, 2014, http://
www.ecology.com/2014/08/25/antidepressant-microbes-soil/; Bonnie L. Grant, "Soil Microbes and Human Health—Learn About the Natural Antidepressant in Soil," 2014, https://
www.gardeningknowhow.com/garden-how-to/soil-fertilizers/antidepressant-microbes
-soil.htm.

CHAPTER 10: CREATING A PROTECTIVE BUBBLE

1. Sandra Blakeslee and Matthew Blakeslee, *The Body Has a Mind of Its Own: How Body Maps in
Your Brain Help You Do (Almost) Everything Better* (New York: Random House, 2007).

2. Judith Orloff, lecture at the Open Center in Manhattan. April 2012.

3. Tinus Smits, http://www.tinussmits.com/3872/vernix-caseosa.aspx.

4. Gurcharan Singh, and G. Archana. 2008. "Unraveling the Mystery of Vernix Caseosa,"
Indian Journal of Dermatology 53, no. 2 (2008): 54, doi:10.4103/0019-5154.41645, https://
www.ncbi.nlm.nih.gov/pmc/articles/PMC2763724/.

5. Tinus Smits, "Inspiring Homeopathy: Vernix Caseosa," http://www.tinussmits.com
/3872/vernix-caseosa.aspx.

6. Personal communication, December 2016.

7. Shimona Tzukernik, "The Kabbalah Coach," https://thekabbalahcoach.com/.

8. Personal communication, July 2017.

CHAPTER 11: REJUVENATING YOUR MOOD WITH COLOR

1. Personal communication, November 11, 2017.

2. Melissa Magsaysay, "Megyn Kelly's Classic Fashion Style," *Los Angeles Times*, March 18, 2012,
accessed 2018, http://www.latimes.com/fashion/alltherage/la-ig-megyn-kelly-20120318
-story.html.

3. "Fashion | Style Guide | What to Wear on Television," Corporate Fashionista, February 21,
2010, accessed 2018, http://www.corporatefashionista.com/what-to-wear-on-tv-5-tips-to
-looking-great/.

Notes

4. Personal communication, January 9, 2017.

5. Stephanie Pappas, "Different Colors Describe Happiness vs. Depression," February 8, 2010, https://www.livescience.com/6084-colors-describe-happiness-depression.html.

6. Jessica Ward Jones, "Decreased Perception of Color in Depression," Psych Central, July 21, 2010, https://psychcentral.com/news/2010/07/21/decreased-perception-of-color -in-depression/15826.html.

7. Niraj Chokshi, "Your Instagram Posts May Hold Clues to Your Mental Health," *New York Times*, August 10, 2017.

8. Oliver Sacks, *An Anthropologist on Mars: Seven Paradoxical Tales* (New York: Vintage, 1996).

9. Kurt Geer, "The Psychology of Colors in Advertising and Marketing," accessed January 2017, http://www.streetdirectory.com/travel_guide/110550/psychology/the_psychology _of_colors_in_advertising_and_marketing.html.

10. "How to Use the Psychology of Colors When Marketing," DashBurst, Small Business Trends, November 2, 2017, https://smallbiztrends.com/2014/06/psychology-of-colors.html.

11. Gregory Ciotti, "The Psychology of Color in Marketing and Branding," *Entrepreneur*, April 13, 2016, https://www.entrepreneur.com/article/233843.

12. "How to Find Your Skin's Undertone," The Blondeshell, March 10, 2014, http://theblondeshell.com/2014/03/10/find-skin-undertone/.

13. Donna Fujii, "Color Analysis: Analyzing Skin Tone, Hair Color, and the Relationship Between Them," *Color with Style*, 2018, http://mailstat.us/tr/t/czigk14aj9j2ssum/u/http://mbeitel.pbworks.com/f/Color+Analysis.pdf.

14. "Johannes Itten 1888–1967," *The Colour Journal*, September 29, 2014, https://thecolourjournal.wordpress.com/2014/09/29/johannes-itten-1888-1967/.

15. Ibid.

16. Ibid.

17. Ibid.

18. Ibid.

19. Rochele H. C. Hirsch, "Suzanne Caygill," Color Designers International, 2018, http://colordesigners.org/suzanne-caygill/.

20. Personal communication, February, 16, 2017.

21. "Image Consultants and Personal Stylist Specialists," House of Colour, 2018, https://www.houseofcolour.co.uk/.

22. "Colours of Sound and Light: Energy, Frequency and Vibration," DK Matai, 2013, http://dkmatai.tumblr.com/post/40378772227/colours-of-sound-and-light-energy-frequency -and.

23. Enoch Tan, "Science of Vibration in Every Aspect of the Physical World," accessed June 2017, http://www.mindreality.com/science-of-vibration-in-every-aspect-of-physical.

24. Personal communication, January 21, 2017.

25. Personal communication, November 8, 2016.

26. Personal communication, May 2017.

CHAPTER 12: YOUR 90-DAY PROGRAM FOR BETTER MOODS

1. Elizabeth Somer. *Food and Mood: The Complete Guide to Eating Well and Feeling Your Best* (New York: Henry Holt, 1995), 135; Richard Wurtman and Judith Wurtman, "Carbohydrates and Depression," *Scientific American*, January 1989, 21–35.

2. Somer, *Food and Mood*, 80.

3. Amanda Salis. "The Science of 'Hangry,' or Why Some People Get Grumpy When They're Hungry," IFLScience, accessed February 5, 2018, iflscience.com/hangry-or-why -some-people-get-grumpy-when-they-re-hungry.

4. Rick Nauert, "Dehydration Influences Mood, Cognition—Part 35037," Psych Central, February 20, 2012, https://psychcentral.com/news/2012/02/20/dehydration-influences -mood-cognition/35037.html/35037; Colin Poltras, "Even Mild Dehydration Can Alter Mood," UConn Today, February 2012, https://today.uconn.edu/2012/02/even-mild -dehydration-can-alter-mood/.

5. "How Antioxidants Can Help Fight Depression," Ecowatch, June 11, 2016, accessed 2018, https://www.ecowatch.com/how-antioxidants-can-help-fight-depression -1891171410.html.

INDEX

Index

anger
  benefits of, 21–22
  bile and, 46
  in Cycle-of-Sanity, 17
  laughter and, 117–118
  valerian for, 82–83
An Anthropologist on Mars (Sacks), 173–174
anxiety
  blue vervain for, 64–65
  chamomile for, 66
  choosing essential oils for, 97
  color and, 172
  fresh milky oats for, 71
  herbal combinations for, 60
  herbs, essential oils, and adaptogens for, 194
  lavender oil for, 93
  lemon balm for, 75
  moods and, 7
  orange oil scent and, 88
  performing random acts of kindness and reduced, 110
  skullcap for, 82
aphrodisiac
  choosing essential oils for, 97
  patchouli oil as, 94
  sandalwood oil as, 96
  See also libido
aromatherapy, 10, 85–104
  choosing a carrier oil, 102–103
  choosing an essential oil, 89–97
  conditioned responses and, 87–88
  how essential oils are made, 89
  how to use essential oils, 98–102
  ingestion of, 102
  overview of, 85–86
  practicing, 191, 192, 193

  quantifiable effect of, 88–89
  side effects of, 104
  who should avoid, 104
  workings of, 86–87
artichoke leaves (*Cynara scolymus*), 46, 49
artificial light, 147
Art Naturals, 89
The Art of Color (Itten), 178
artwork in the bedroom, 151
ashwagandha root (*Withania somnifera*), 54
Asian ginseng root (*Panax ginseng*), 54
aspirin, 42
associative learning, essential oils and, 88
asthma, as contraindication for aromatherapy, 104
Aura Cacia, 89
autumn, in color analysis, 179, 180
avocado oil, 102
awareness, gaining control of moodiness through, 8, 10
awareness practice, 166

Back to Eden (Kloss), 11
bacopa (*Brahmi monnier*), 63–64
base notes, 90
basil oil, 90
bath
  essential oils to add to, 101–102
  essential oils to avoid, 98
bathroom, balancing energy in, 153
bedroom
  artwork in, 151
  limiting use of electronics in, 151
  organize what's under your bed, 150
  placement of bed, 150
  rearranging, 191
  rose quartz in, 153

Index

Index

Index

helping control moods and, 7, 8

homeopathic, 24

for specific emotions, 194

to support the liver, 42–43, 48–51

See also mood herbs

"Herbs at a Glance" website, 58

Herbs Etc., 61

Herbs for Stress & Anxiety (Gladstar), 203

Herbs for Women's Health (Bove), 45

Herbs of Light, 61

Herz, Rachel S., 87–88

high blood pressure, as contraindication for aromatherapy, 104. *See also* blood pressure

Hindu holidays, full moon and, 135

Hippocrates, 41

holy basil (*Ocimum tenuiflorum, O. Sanskrit, O. gratissumum*), 55, 71–73

home

artwork in the bedroom, 151

bathroom, 153

corners and, 152

decluttering, 149–150

flowers in, 148–149

free-flowing water in, 152

front door, 147

houseplants in, 148

light in, 147–148

limiting use of electronics in the bedroom, 151

organizing under the bed, 150

placement of bed, 150

removing shoes at front door, 151

repairing objects in, 149

rose quartz in, 153

rule of pairs and, 149

scent, 153

shapes in, 152

soft edges and, 152

use of color, 151

using mirrors with purpose in, 152

homeopathic remedies, 24–25

homeopathy, 9

overview, 24–25

homeopathy training, 12

houseplants

in the bathroom, 153

in the home, 148

hunger, 199–200

hydration, 200

hydrosols, 89

hypothalamus, stress and, 43

immune system

laughter and, 117

smiling and, 114

incense, 153

ingestion of essential oils, 102

insight, happiness and, 18–19

insomnia

California poppy for, 65

chamomile for, 66

choosing essential oils for, 97

herbal combinations for, 60

herbs, essential oils, and adaptogens for, 194

kava kava for, 73–74

passion flower for, 77–78

skullcap for, 82

valerian for, 83

wild lettuce for, 83

Inspiring Homeopathy (Smits), 163–164

interest, listening intuitively and showing, 129

Index

Index

liver
  bitters and, 47, 49
  "cleansing" or "detoxifying," 45–46
  effect of stress on, 44, 47–48
  reasons to support the, 44–48
  symptoms of congested, 48
liver support herbs, 42–43, 48–51, 190,
    192
  quick reference guide to, 195
longevity, laughter and, 118
Los Angeles Times (newspaper), 170
lotus flower, 149
Louv, Richard, 153
love, mimosa bark and, 76–77
low blood sugar, 199
lucky bamboo, 148
lying, signals person may be, 133

Maimonides, 41–42
Majeski, Shloma, 118
Man's Search for Meaning (Frankl), 118
Manyasi, 52
Marder, Gwen, 170
marjoram oil, 95
Masé, Guido, 46, 47
massage, essential oil, 100–101
master herbalist RH (AHG), author as, 9
Materia Medica, 25–26
Mayer, Emeran, 124
meadowsweet, 42
medications
  herbs as alternative to mood-related, 9
  interaction of essential oils with, 104
meditation
  creating protective bubble and, 161–162
  quieting the mind and, 129–130
melancholy
  defined, 17

social withdrawal and, 22
  See also depression; sadness
memory
  emotional, 27
  rosemary for, 80
  rosemary oil for, 95
menstrual cycle, chasteberry for irregular,
    66, 67
The Method program, 166–167
middle notes, 90
Mie University School of Medicine (Japan),
    88
milk thistle seed (*Silybum marianum*), 50–51
mimosa bark (*Albizia julibrissin*), 76–77
mind, quieting the, 129–130
mind-body connection, Hippocrates and, 41
The Mind-Gut Connection (Mayer), 124
mirrors, use with purpose in home, 152
Miyazaki, Yoshifumi, 154
Monell Chemical Senses Center, 88
money plant, 148
The Monographs (Commission E), 58
Montgomery, Pam, 70
mood herbs, 59–84
  adult dosages, 61–62
  children's dosages, 62
  how to begin using, 58–59
  how to take, 61
  safety of, 58–59
  sources for, 61
  working with herbalist, 59–61
moodiness, 7
  awareness of, 8
  common essential oils used for, 90–97
moods
  charting, 33–38, 197–198
  color and, 172–174
  effect of exercise on, 23

235

Index

Index

Index

Index

ABOUT THE AUTHORS

SARA-CHANA SILVERSTEIN is a master herbalist RH (AHG), classical homeopath, board-certified lactation consultant (IBCLC), businesswoman, wife, keynote speaker, and mother of seven children. She is regularly featured on TV news shows across the United States, discussing how people can integrate alternative with conventional medicine. She is a consultant to many pediatricians, surgeons, obstetricians, midwives, and general doctors, and is currently guest lecturing to residents at New York medical schools. She wrote and developed the app "Sara-Chana's Savvy Breastfeeding Guide."

Sara-Chana grew up in Los Angeles, California, as a precocious, high-energy child with an inquiring mind. At age five, she became an actress, appearing in national commercials, TV shows, and film. Simultaneously she was a gymnast, competing at national and international levels. She was an AAU Junior Olympic champion. She seized the opportunity and was given a costarring role in *Nadia*, a major motion picture about the Olympic champion, Romanian gymnast Nadia Comaneci.

Despite evidence to the contrary—her intense acting career and sports activities—her real childhood dream was to become a writer and to attend medical school. After she graduated from UC Irvine, she was invited through Yale School of Drama to spend a summer at Oxford University in England to study Shakespeare. True confession? Most of her time was spent in the Oxford library, reading books about herbs and not Shakespeare. With apologies to Will.

Upon returning to Los Angeles, her research into herbs and their healing properties quickly accelerated. Once she moved to New York, she opened a clinic where she practiced as a lactation consultant, master herbalist, and homeopathy practitioner. Her waiting room quickly filled with women and their husbands, children, and grandparents all wanting herbs to help them better achieve health.

SUSAN K. GOLANT, MA, is a writer specializing in bio-psych-social topics. She has coauthored and ghostwritten more than forty books on health, emotional well-being, spirituality, parenting, and women's issues, including three books on mental health with former First Lady Rosalynn Carter. She lives in Los Angeles with her husband, psychologist Dr. Mitch Golant.